SUP

JN036940

診

技師のための

医療英語

順天堂大学 保健医療学部
診療放射線学科 特任教授 **坂野康昌**

南 山 堂

序

　日本国内において，病院の診療放射線科は，院内の各種診療科の中でも全診療科対応の部門のひとつといえる．つまり，小児科・婦人科・外科・内科・救急外来などすべての診療科に対応した検査診断や治療を実施する科なのである．また，近時，外国人患者も激増しており，世界共通語ともいえる英語を用いたコミュニケーション能力が求められる場面は病院内でも多くなっている．

　このため，英語での略語や専門用語の飛び交う状況にある医療環境にあって，各科の専門的な検査治療の内容に応じた知識と患者接遇が不可欠となっている．こうした医療現場における状況を打開し，良好な患者対応をするためのツールとして，実践的な書籍を作成した．

　日本の診療放射線技師は，所定の教育を修了し，国家試験合格後のライセンス取得により診断・核医学・放射線治療の3部門すべてで活躍できる．もちろん専門性向上のため日々の研鑽を続けながらではあるが，世界的に比較しても，この資格はまさにスペシャリストとジェネラリストを兼ね備えたスーパーテクノロジストと言っても過言ではない．現状において，検査や治療の専門用語は英語が標準であり，専門用語の略語も日常的に使用されている．こうした部門であるからこそ，自らの担当業務における語彙力と患者接遇における語彙力を融合させていく必要がある．

また，学会発表や遠隔での国際カンファレンス実施の際にも共通語としての英語での会話となり，国内外の研究会や学会においても英語での発表が通常化している時代となった.

　もう日本人は英語が"下手"だからというだけで，現状から回避できる理由にはならないことを強く認識しなくてはならない. アジアの諸外国を見回しても，各国に母国語があり，この点では日本の状況と同様であるが，その他に一般学習や専門学習のために使用するテキストは英語版を使用しており，彼らは日常会話にも良い意味で語学を反映させ，努力を続けていることを重視すべきである.

　日本の専門書は日本語のみで書かれるものが多く，日本人が専門性を高める学修には非常に優れている. しかし，国際性に乏しくなっていることも否定できない. こうした間隙を埋め，この状況を打破し，更なる努力によって新たな扉を開いていくために本書を活用していただきたい.

　2021 年 1 月

坂野康昌

目　次

一般撮影編

□ 放射線科　radiology department
□ X 線検査部門　X-ray examination department
□ X 線撮影装置　X-ray apparatus
□ 電子カルテ　electronic medical chart／electrical health
　record／electronic patient chart

A scenario for the foreign patient

1. Changing room

2. Positioning

3. Instruction and Signal

4. Greeting

5. Encouragement‼ Cheer up!

Useful expression

Removing your clothes is very important in this examination because it can help us to have a better image of your abdomen.

Do not worry about it because it is not a dangerous examination. I am here to assist you carefully.

Today, we are going to have chest X-ray test. So, please take off your upper clothes.

Today, we are going to have abdominal X-ray. So, could you please take off everything including your underwear and change into the hospital gown?

I am here to assist you. Please stay calm. Do not worry.

If you need any help, please let me know as soon as possible.

Please take a deep breath and hold it.

Please inhale deeply and hold it.

Please exhale and hold it.

Please keep this position.

Please stay still.

You can now relax.

Relax your muscles and breathing.

You did a good job today!

The X-ray examination has been completed.

Thank you for your cooperation.

Take care of yourself.

I wish you a fast recovery.

The examination found no health issues.

After looking at your medical findings we found no reason to worry.

You are completely fine.

The examination ended well.

Your tests came out fine.

あなたの名前を確認させてください.

> Let me confirm your name.

毎回チェックしていますので，ご自身でお名前と誕生日をおっしゃっていただけますか？

> Can you verify your name and DOB for me, please? (DOB: date of birth)

> Can you tell me your name and DOB?

> Since I check the patient every time, could you give me your name and DOB?

□ 患者確認　identify a patient and to prevent a wrong patient

こんにちは．私があなたのX線撮影伝票を受け取ります.

> Hello. Would you please give me your medical form for the X-ray test?

> Hello. May I have your medical form for the X-ray test, please?

□ medical form／voucher：いずれも医師から受け取る用紙 (the piece of paper you got from the doctor)

X線検査の前に，あなたの妊娠の有無を確認させてください.

> I need to confirm if you are possibly pregnant.

> I have a question before X-ray. Is there a chance you are pregnant right now?

胎児に影響があるといけませんので，X線検査の前に妊娠の確認をしています．

> Because the radiation has a negative effect on babies, I would like to confirm your pregnancy before this X-ray examination.

> Before this X-ray examination, I need to confirm if you are possibly pregnant as the radiation is not good for the baby.

> Before you undergo the X-ray, I just need to confirm if you are pregnant right now because it may harm the baby.

 放射線が怖いのですが，大丈夫でしょうか？ 痛いですか？

> I am worried about radiation. Is it safe? Do I feel pain?

> I am afraid of radiation. Is it safe for me? Does it hurt or not?

> A radiation is scary for me. Will it be all right? Do I really have no pain?

> I am a bit scared of the radiation. Is it all right? Do I feel pain?

ご心配なく．大丈夫ですよ．落ち着いてくださいね．

> Do not worry. Please be calm.

> Do not worry. You are all right.

> You do not have to worry. Please stay calm.

私たちがしっかり対応しますから大丈夫ですよ．心配しないでください．

We will take good care of you. Do not worry.

I am here for you. I am here to assist you. It is no problem.

もし助けが必要でしたらすぐに知らせてくださいね．

If you need any help, please let me know as soon as possible.

Please tell me as soon as possible if you need any help.

放射線の量は微量なので，健康には問題ありません．

The X-ray is only a very small amount of radiation, so it will not affect your health.

The X-ray is only a very small amount of radiation, so it will not hurt you anyway.

（患者）入院中，毎日のように CT 検査や X 線検査をしていました．健康に影響はありませんか？

I had CT-scan and X-ray examination every day while I was in the hospital. Did they affect my health?

あなたに健康被害を与えるような被曝には到底及びませんので心配はいりません．

You do not have to worry because you will not be exposed to radiation that may affect your health.

お名前をお呼びするまで2番と書かれた部屋の前で少々お待ちください．

> Please wait in front of the room number 2 until your name is called.

> Please wait a few minutes in front of the room No.2 till I call your name.

ブッシュさん，更衣室にお入りください．

> Mr. Bush, please come into the changing room. 男性

> Madam / Ms. Bush, please come into the changing room. 女性（既婚／未婚）

X線検査のために衣服を脱いでください．

> Please remove your clothes to take the X-ray examination.

> Please take off your clothes for this X-ray examination.

胸部のX線写真を撮りますので，下着をとって上半身裸になってください．

> Please undress from the waist up because I will take your X-ray examination.

> You will undergo the X-ray, so please take off your clothes from the waist up.

胸部のX線検査をしますので，このガウンに着替えてください．

> You will undergo your chest X-ray, so please change into this hospital gown.

You will undergo the chest X-ray examination, so please change into this gown.

Please change into this gown, because I will take your chest X-ray.

患者 なぜ X 線検査のために服を脱ぐ必要があるのですか？

Why do I need to undress for the X-ray examination?

Why do I have to take off my clothes for the X-ray examination?

Why should I take off my clothes during the X-ray examination?

ボタンや金属が X 線画像の中に写り込み，正常画像の妨げになります．

Buttons and metals come out in X-ray results and affect the normal images.

We do not want to get inaccurate X-ray results because a button and metal will influence the examination.

ボタンや金属があるようでしたら，シャツと下着を脱いでください．

Please remove your shirt and your underwear if these have any buttons and metals.

Please take off your shirt and your underwear which attached any buttons and metals.

義歯などはこの検査（正常画像）の妨げになります．

Your denture will affect this examination.

Wearing false teeth will influence this examination.

☐ 義歯 denture／artificial teeth／dental plate

（患者）放射線は見えないからなおさら怖いのです．

Since I can't see the radiation, I feel much scary.

I feel more fear because I can't see the radiation.

全然痛いことはありません．心配しないで大丈夫です．

There is no pain. Please do not worry.

It does not hurt at all, please do not worry.

こちらへどうぞ．X線防護用の鉛入り前掛けを着用いただきますね．

This way, please. Please wear the lead-apron of the X-ray protector.

This way, please. Would you wear this lead-apron of the X-ray protective shield?

あなたの胸部の正面写真（P-A）を撮ります．
（P-A：posterior-anterior）

We will begin this procedure of P-A (posterior-anterior). I will take your chest X-ray now.

We will begin this procedure of P-A (posterior-anterior). You undergo the chest X-ray examination now.

ここにあなたの顎を乗せてください．（P-A）

Please put your chin on this area.

Please carry your chin on board here.

両腕でこの辺りを抱え込むようにしてください．

Please put both your arms around here.

Please set your arms on this area.

このままの姿勢で動かないでください．

Please hold this position and do not move.

Please keep this position and hold it.

Please do not move for keeping the same position.

そのままで，しばらくの間（5秒間）動かないでください．

Do not move for a while, please.

Please do not move for five seconds.

患者さんに協力していただく指示や合図があります．

There are instructions and signals that require the patient's cooperation.

There are instructions and signals which need the patient's cooperation.

深く息を吸ってください．

Please take a deep breath.

Inhale deeply, please.

Would you please inhale deeply? 丁寧な表現

Could you please take a deep breath? 丁寧な表現

腹部の X 線検査を受けてください．
腹部の X 線写真（KUB）を撮ります．

You will undergo abdominal X-ray examination.
I will take the X-ray of your abdomen (KUB).

KUB とは腎臓・輸尿管・膀胱の略語です．

KUB stands for kidney, ureter, and bladder.

KUB is the abbreviation of kidney, ureter, and bladder.

息を大きく吸い込んで，そのまま止めてください．

Take a deep breath and hold it, please.

Please inhale and hold it.

Breathe in deeply and hold it. Stay still, please.

Would you please take a deep breath and hold it? 丁寧な表現

私の方を向いてください．今度は側面からの X 線写真を撮ります．（R-L）

Can you turn toward me? I take the lateral X-ray photograph this time.

I take the lateral X-ray photograph from the side this time. (R-L)

両腕を挙げてください．

Please raise both your arms.

このままの姿勢でいてください.

Please keep this position.

Please try not to move.

Try not to move.

X線検査台の上に横になってください.

Please lie on the X-ray examination table.

Please lie down on the X-ray examination table.

息を吐いてください.

Breathe out, please.

Please exhale.

Would you please exhale deeply? 丁寧な表現

Could you please breathe out? 丁寧な表現

最初に息を吸い込んで, それから息を吐きだして, そのまま止めてください.

Please inhale first and then breathe out and hold it.

Please inhale first and then exhale completely and hold it.

その他の合図

腹ばい（うつぶせ）に寝てください.（腹臥位）

Please lie on your stomach.

Please lie face down.

仰向け（上向き）に寝てください．（仰臥位）

Please lie on your back.

Please lie face up.

うつぶせに寝てください．それから次は仰向けに寝てください．（回転）

Lie face down. Then lie face up.

Lie on your stomach and then lie on your back.

右側を下にして横向きに寝てください．（側臥位）

Please lie on your right side.

Please lie down on your right side.

左側を下にして横向きに寝てください．（側臥位）

Please lie on your left side.

Please lie down on your left side.

☐ 腹臥位　prone position
☐ 仰臥位　supine position
☐ 側臥位　lateral position

はい，検査が終わりました．呼吸を楽にしてください．楽にしてください．

> It is all right, the examination is over. Please relax your breathing. You can relax now.

> All right, the examination has been completed. Please relax your muscles. You can now relax.

はい，（呼吸を）楽にしてください．

> All right, relax breathing, please.

> Please relax your breathing.

> You can now relax.

寒いですから早く服を着てください．

> Please put on your clothes quickly because it is cold.

> Because you feel cold, please wear clothes as soon as possible.

（患者）**どうもありがとう，この後はどこへ行けば（何をすれば）いいのですか？**

> Thank you. Where should I go to next?

> Thanks a lot. What should I do next?

説明いたしますから，それまで座ってお待ちください．

> Let me explain it. Please have a seat until then.

次に内科で診察があります．お声がけしますから，受付で少しお待ちください．

> Next, the attending doctor consult you at the internal medicine department.
>
> Please have a seat in the waiting area near reception until I call your name.

（患者）ご協力感謝します．／ありがとうございます．

> Thank you for your help.
>
> Thanks for your cooperation.
>
> Thank you for your kind assistance.

ご協力感謝します．

> Thank you for your cooperation.
>
> I appreciate to your cooperation.

お大事に！

> Please take care of yourself.
>
> I hope you will be better soon.
>
> I hope you get better soon.
>
> I wish you a fast recovery.

Supplement

一般的にいうと，いくつかの放射線検査には副作用があります．

Generally speaking, some radiation examination have side effects.

放射線はときに皮膚に紅斑や皮膚炎（過敏症）を引き起こします．

The radiation sometimes cause erythema or dermatitis (irritation) to your skin.

☐ 皮膚の紅斑　erythema
☐ 皮膚炎　dermatitis
☐ 炎症／過敏症　irritation

高線量の放射線は男性の性腺（生殖腺）に障害を与えます．

High amount of radiation dose can damage male gonads.

放射線の早期障害の一つには脱毛があります．

One of the early damages due to radiation is hair loss.

☐ 損傷　damage
☐ 障害　disorder

放射線の後発障害には白内障があります．

The late disorder due to radiation is a cataract.

一般撮影の部門では, 必要最小限の放射線量で撮影するため, 患者さんの放射線による影響や副作用については心配いりません.

In the general radiography department, the radiographs are taken with the minimum necessary radiation dose, so there is no need to worry about the effects and side effects of radiation on patients.

泣き止まない子どもの X 線撮影では保護者の協力を必要とする場合があります.

Parental assistance may be required for X-rays of children who cannot stop crying.

保護者には防護用の鉛入りエプロンを着用していただき, 子どもから顔が見えるところにいてもらいます.

Parents are required to wear protective lead-in aprons and to be in a place where their children can see the faces.

胸部の一般 X 線撮影の方向の指示は「P → A」や「R → L」で示されます.

The direction of chest X-ray photography is indicated by "P → A" or "R → L."

「P → A」や「R → L」の意味は, 後→前, 右→左です.

"P → A" or "R → L" means posterior-anterior (back-front), right-left.

白血病は血液や骨髄のがんのことです．

> Leukemia is a cancer of the blood or bone marrow.

この患者さんはウイルスや細菌や寄生虫に感染しやすいです．

> This patient is susceptible to viruses, bacteria, and parasites.

☐ ウイルス　viruses
☐ 細菌　bacteria／germs
☐ 病原体　pathogen

佐藤さんは高血圧のために眩暈（めまい）があります．

> Ms. Sato has vertigo due to her high blood pressure.

☐ 眩暈（めまい）　vertigo／dizziness

どこが痛みますか？

> Where does it hurt?
>
> Where do you feel the pain?

どのような痛みですか？

> What kind of pain?
>
> What is your pain like?

どのような痛みか説明してくれますか？

> Could you describe your pain to me?

鋭い痛みまたは鈍痛のどちらですか？

Which do you feel, sharp or dull pain?

- ☐ 鋭い痛み a sharp pain
- ☐ 鈍い痛み a dull pain
- ☐ 締めつけるような痛み a squeezing pain
- ☐ 拍動性のずきずきする痛み a pulsating pain

② 造影透視編

☐ 胃透視　upper gastrointestinal tract radiography
　(upper GI)
☐ 注腸検査　lower gastrointestinal tract radiography
　(lower GI)

胃透視

検査前に，いくつか確認させてください．

> Before this examination, I would like to ask a few questions.
>
> There are a few things we should verify before the test.
>
> There are a few things that I would like to confirm before the examination.

バリウム検査を以前にも受けたことがありますか？

> Have you experienced this barium examination before?
>
> Have you undergone this barium (solution) examination before?

検査のため，朝食はとっていませんね？

> Do you keep fasting for this examination now?

食べ物が胃に残っていると，十分な検査（造影透視）ができません．

> If you eat anything, we will not be able to get a good X-ray result.

> When food is left in your stomach, enough examination is not possible.

> If you have leftover food in your stomach, we cannot get clear images of your organs.

検査台に足跡が描いてあります．

> Footprints are drawn on the examination stand.

> Footprints are marked on the examination base.

> There is an outline for your feet on the examination stand.

そこに立っていただけますか？

> Please stand there.

> Could you stand there?

この白い液体はバリウムといいます．

> This white liquid is called barium solution.

> This is a cup of barium solution.

造影剤というもので胃の検査に必要です．

> The gastric examination needs this contrast agent.

> This is a contrast material which is necessary for gastric examination.

消化器系の検査で使うバリウムという造影剤は検査後に大便とともに排泄されます.

> The contrast agent called barium solution which used in the digestive system examination is excreted with stool after the examination.

□ 造影剤　contrast agent／contrast material／contrast media

それでは, これから造影検査(透視検査)を行います.(食道造影)

> Now, we will begin the barium drinking test.
>
> Now, we will start the barium swallowing examination.

最初は飲み込まずに, バリウム(白い液体)を1口だけ口の中に溜めてください.(嚥下試験)

> Let it stay in your mouth for a while. I will instruct you when to swallow it.
>
> Please put the barium inside your mouth and do not swallow it yet.
>
> First, take a sip and let it stay in your mouth, and do not swallow it yet.
>
> First, take a sip of the barium solution and let it stay in your mouth, and do not swallow it yet.

担当医などの合図に従ってバリウムを飲んでください.

> Swallow the barium upon the instruction of the doctor or person in charge.
>
> Wait for the instruction of the doctor or person in charge to swallow it.

バリウムをまず1口飲んでください.

First, drink (swallow) one sip of barium solution.

そのまま動かないでください.

Please stay still there.

Please do not move and keep this position.

カップの中のバリウムを1口飲み込んで,動かないでいてください.

Drink only a sip of barium solution in the cup, and please do not move.

カップのバリウムを2口ほど飲み込んでください.

Please swallow approximately two sips of barium in the cup.

Please drink two sips of barium in the cup.

Please swallow two sips of barium solution from the cup.

1口バリウムを飲み込んで5秒後にバリウムを2口ほど飲み込んでください.

Drink 1 sip of barium solution, and after 5 seconds you can sip approximately 1 to 2 sips of barium solution.

次に，この顆粒（発泡剤）を少量の水で素早く飲み込んでください．
［海外では発泡剤を使用しない場合も多く，理解を得るため説明を要す．］

> Next, swallow immediately the granulated medicine with a small amount of water.

> Next, swallow the granules (foaming agent) followed by a small sip of water as soon as possible.

> Next, swallow the granules (foaming agent) followed by a small amount of water immediately.

これは胃を膨らませるために必要です．胃を大きく膨らませるために飲んでいただきたいのです．そうすることで検査で胃が見やすくなります．すぐに飲み込んでください．

> This is necessary to puff out your stomach. You need to drink it so that your stomach will puff out greatly. Then we could easily see it by examination. Please swallow it immediately.

バリウム（造影剤）を私の合図に合わせて飲み込んでください．

> Please drink barium solution by my indication.

> Please swallow barium solution (contrast media) by my signal.

カップの中の残りのバリウムを全部飲んでください．

> Please drink up all barium solution in the cup.

> Please swallow all remaining barium in the cup.

そのままの姿勢で動かないでください．

    Now, please keep that position.

    Stay like that, please.

    Stay still, please.

    Do not move, please.

はい，楽にしてください．

    All right, try to relax.

    You can relax now.

    You can now relax.

Ｘ線検査台の上に寝てください．

    Please lie on the X-ray examination table.

    Please lie down on the X-ray examination table.

仰向け（上向き）に寝てください．（仰臥位）

    Please lie on your back.

    Please lie face up.

腹ばい（うつぶせ）に寝てください．（腹臥位）

    Please lie on your stomach.

    Please lie face down.

右側を下にして横向きに寝てください．（側臥位）

    Please lie on your right side.

    Lie down on your right side.

    Please lie down on the bed on your right side.

左側を下にして横向きに寝てください．（側臥位）

Please lie on your left side.

Please lie down on your left side.

☐ 仰臥位　supine position
☐ 腹臥位　prone position
☐ 側臥位　lateral position

右の方から腹ばいになってください（ぐるりと回ります）．

Turn to your right, lie on your stomach.

Please lay on your stomach from the right.
(Turning to right)

左の方から腹ばいになってください（ぐるりと回ります）．

Turn to your left, lie on your stomach.

Please lay on your stomach from the left.
(Turning to left)

腹ばいから仰向けになるようにして寝てください（ぐるりと回ります）．

You need to lie down on your stomach and then lie down on your back.

両脇の手すりを握ってください．頭が下がります．

Please hold on to the bars beside you. Your head will be lowered.

Hold on to the both side handles. Your head will go down.

お腹で息を吸ってください.

Breathe in your stomach.

Breathe in your abdomen.

深く息を吸って，横隔膜を広げてください.（吸気）

Take a deep breath and let your diaphragm expand.

息を吐いてください.

Breathe out.

Could you exhale?

お腹（の動き）を止めていてください.

Please keep your abdomen still.

Please stop your abdomen from breathing.

楽にしてください.

Relax, please.

You can now relax.

Try to relax your breathing, please.

X 線装置と検出器の間に X 線撮影する腹部の部分を慎重に配置するように位置決めします.

The part of your abdomen to be X-rayed will be positioned carefully between the X-ray machine and the detector.

正encased。

求められる X 線像に応じて，立ち上がる，台の上に寝る，または横になるようにお願いする場合があります．

> You may be asked to stand up, lie flat, or lie on your side on a table, depending on the X-ray view your healthcare provider has asked for.

造影透視編

装置（検査台）が水平になります．

> This apparatus moves horizontally.（立位から水平へ）

> This examination table elevate horizontally.（低頭位から水平へ）

お顔を右側に向けてください．

> Turn your face to your right.

> Turn your head to the right.

そちらから（右側から）回転して仰向けに戻ります．

> You will turn upward from your right side.

> Turn to the right, onto your back.

台が動きます．じっとしていてください．

> Please stay still as the examination table moves.

> The examination table will move now. Please remain still.

右腰をひねって少し上げてください．

> Turn your right waist upward.

> Can you twist and adjust your right waist upward?

> Could you twist your right waist and lift it upward.

今度は逆に，左腰を上げてください．

> Now to the left, please. The other way, lift up your left waist.

> Now, the other side. Can you twist your left waist slightly?

> Could you twist your left waist and lift it upward?.

体を右に2回，回転してください．

> Please rotate your body to the right side twice.

> Please turn your body to the right twice.

元の姿勢（仰向け）に戻って結構です．

> All right, you can return to your original position.

> You can go back to lying on your back.

> You can go back to the original position by lying on your back.

複数の位置からX線を撮影する場合があります．

> You may have X-rays taken from more than one position.

頭が下がります．（寝台が逆傾斜する場合の指示）

> Your head will tilt down.

> We are going to lower the position of your head now.

横の手すりをしっかりと握っていてください.

> Grip the side bars tightly, please.
>
> Hold on to the handles on the side, please.

頭が上がってきます.両足を台にしっかりと付けてください.

> Your head will be tilted up. Please attach both feet to the stand well.
>
> Your head will elevate now. Keep your feet on the pedestal.

検査台が立ってきます.

> The examining table will move in upright position.
>
> You are going to back to the standing position.

お疲れさまでした.

> You did a good job there.
>
> Thank you for your cooperation today.

あなたの検査は全部終わりました.

> Your procedure has been completed.
>
> All your examinations are over (with).
>
> (over with は米口語)

今日は水分をたくさん摂ってください.

> Try to drink lots of fluid today.
>
> Please drink a lot of water today.

下剤を差し上げますので，自宅に戻られてからお飲みください．

> I will give you laxatives, so swallow them once when you get home.

> You will receive a laxative. Please swallow it when you get home.

翌日か翌々日あたりに便が白くなります．問題ありません．心配なさらないでください．

> Your stools may appear white for the next day or the day after tomorrow. No problem. Do not worry, please.

注腸検査

これから大腸の検査を始めます．

> Now, we will start your large intestinal examination.

肛門からバリウムと空気を注入します．

> We will inject barium solution and air into your anus.

> You will undergo the enema of barium solution and air.

> We are going to pass a mixture of barium solution, water, and air into your colon through a tube.

お腹が張ってきますが，心配いりません．

Your stomach will inflate a little, but do not worry.

You may feel some pressure in your stomach, but it is nothing to worry about.

台の上で，こちら側へぐるぐると３回ほど回っていただきます．

On the table you will turn (to your right / left) three times.

Turn over this way three times, please.

これは腸壁に造影剤をよく付けるためです．

This is to let the contrast agent coat the intestine walls.

This is to help the barium thoroughly coat the lining of your colon.

あなたのそばにいますから，つらくなったら私に教えてください．

Because I am near you, please tell me if you feel bad.

Please talk me if you feel sick, since I am beside you.

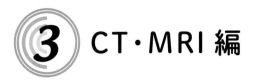

③ CT・MRI 編

☐ コンピュータ断層撮影　computed tomography（CT）
☐ 磁気共鳴映像法　magnetic resonance imaging（MRI）

午前中に造影CT検査がある方は, 朝食を摂らないでください.

> If you take a contrast enhancement CT scan in the morning, do not eat breakfast.

> If you undergo a contrast enhancement CT examination in the morning, you need fasting.

> If you take a contrast enhancement CT scan in the morning, do not eat breakfast because you need to fast.

午後に造影CT検査がある方は, 朝食を9時までに摂り, 昼食は摂らないでください.

> If you have a contrast enhancement CT scan in the afternoon, please have breakfast by 9:00AM and do not have lunch.

検査着に着替えていただく場合がありますので, 着替えやすい服装で来院してください.

> You may need to change into hospital gown, so please wear clothes that are easy to change.

> You will be instructed to change clothes during the test, so kindly wear clothes that are easy to change.

検査時にはネックレス・湿布薬・金具の付いた下着類ははずしてください．

Please remove necklaces, poultice, and underwear included metal fittings at the time of examination.

緊急の患者さんの検査が発生する場合がありますので，その際にはあなたの予約検査時間がずれる場合があります．

There are times when an urgent patient's examination occurs, so your appointment time may be shifted.

Sudden CT-examinations are sometimes necessary to urgent patient, so please cooperate with change on this case.

（今日は）どうされましたか？

What brings you here today?

What brings you to see me today?

How can I help you today?

What can I do for you today?

 CT と MRI の検査をするように主治医から言われました．

My doctor told me to undergo CT and MRI examinations.

わかりました，私は CT と MRI 担当の診療放射線技師で徳川秀吉と申します．

I see, I am Hideyoshi Tokugawa, a radiological technologist in charge of CT and MRI.

本日のあなたの CT と MRI 検査について説明させてください.

> Let me explain about your CT and MRI examination.

CT や MRI は画像診断に非常に役に立ちます.

> CT scan or MRI exam can be very useful for imaging diagnosis.

MRI と CT とでは類似点と相違点があります.

> There are similarities and differences between MRI and CT scan.

MRI は強力な超電導磁石と RF 波を使い,CT は X 線を使って撮像しています.

> MRI uses powerful superconducting magnets and RF waves, but CT scan is captured using X-rays.

CT のほうが出血病変などに対する感度はより高く,MRI は脳梗塞・脳腫瘍・後頭蓋窩(脳幹付近)の診断により適しています.

> CT scan is more sensitive to bleeding lesions, but MRI is better for cerebral infarction, brain tumor, and the posterior fossa (near the brain stem).

☐ 脳血管疾患　cerebral vascular disease
☐ 脳梗塞　cerebral infarction
☐ 脳挫傷　cerebral contusion
☐ 脳卒中　cerebral apoplexy／stroke

CT 検査

患者さんの取り違え防止のため，お名前と生年月日をおっしゃっていただけますか．

> Please state your name and date of birth to avoid mistaking you for other patients.

> Please give me your name and date of birth to prevent you from being confused with other patients.

CT 検査の前に本人確認のためお名前と生年月日をおっしゃっていただけますか．

> Please give me your name and date of birth to confirm your identity before CT.

> Please tell me your name and date of birth to verify your identity before CT.

CT は X 線を用いて身体の輪切りの断層画像を作り，病気の診断に役立てる検査です．

> CT is an examination that makes sliced images of the body by using X-rays to help diagnosis of diseases.

CT 検査は造影剤を使用する場合と使用しない場合の 2 種類の検査があります．

> There are two types of CT examinations, one with and without a contrast agent.

□ 造影剤　contrast agent／contrast material

（造影剤を使用しない）単純 CT 検査の撮影時間は約 5〜10 分です.

> Imaging time for simple CT examination (without using contrast agent) is about 5 to 10 minutes.

（造影剤を使用する）造影 CT 検査の撮影時間は約 15〜30 分です.

> Imaging time for contrast CT scan (using a contrast medium) is about 15 to 30 minutes.

検査部位の違いによって検査時間も異なります.

> The test time also differs depending on the examination region.
>
> The examination time also varies depending on the test part.

造影 CT 検査では，病気の存在を正確に診断するために非イオン性ヨード造影剤を静脈内に注射します.

> In contrast CT examination, a nonionic iodine contrast agent is injected intravenously in order to accurately diagnose the presence of a disease.

静脈注射時は血管に沿ってわずかな熱感が現れ，体が温かくなってきます.

> During intravenous injection, a slight sensation of heat appears along the blood vessels, your body will be warm.

ごくまれに造影剤に対する副作用が出現することがあります.

Side effects of contrast agents may appear very rarely.

□ 造影剤の副作用
軽い副作用（発生頻度 0.1〜5％以下）：蕁麻疹, くしゃみ,
吐き気, 嘔吐, めまい, かゆみ, など
重い副作用（発生頻度 約 0.2％）：血圧低下, 呼吸困難, 意
識障害, など

副作用の軽度の症状には，蕁麻疹，くしゃみ，吐き気，嘔吐，
めまい，かゆみなどがあります.

Symptoms of mild side effects include urticaria, sneezing, nausea, vomiting, dizziness, and itching.

軽い副作用の発生頻度は 0.1〜5％以下です.

The frequency of mild side effects is 0.1 to 5% or less.

深刻な副作用の症状は, 血圧低下, 呼吸困難, 意識障害などです.

Symptoms of serious side effects include decreased blood pressure, dyspnea, and impaired consciousness.

重い副作用の発生頻度は約 0.2％程度です.

The frequency of serious side effects is approximately 0.2%.

造影 CT 検査後には，使用したヨード造影剤は尿から体外へ排出されますので，普段よりできるだけ水分を多めにお取りください．

> After contrast CT examination, the used iodine contrast agent is excreted from the body through urine, so please take as much water as possible than usual.

こちらへどうぞ．この寝台に仰向けで寝て（横たわって）ください．楽にしてください．

> This way, please. Please lie on your back on this bed. Please relax.

このままの姿勢で動かないでください．

> Please stay like that. Please hold that position.
>
> Please stay still. Please keep that position.
>
> Kindly stay still.

これから CT 検査をしていきますが，向こう側からの私の呼吸の合図に従ってください．

> I will perform CT scan of your abdomen, so please follow my breathing cues from over there.
>
> Let me take CT scan of your abdomen, so please follow my breathing cues from over there.

息を大きく吸い込んで，そのまま止めてください．

> Take a deep breath and hold it.
>
> Inhale deeply and hold it.

Breathe in deeply and hold it.

息を大きく吐いて，そのまま止めてください．

Exhale completely and stay still like that.

Breathe out completely and stay still.

どうぞ呼吸を楽にしてください．楽にしてください．

Relax please. You can now relax.

Relax your breathing and muscles.

You can now relax.

楽にしてください．CT 検査は終わりました．

Please relax. The CT examination is over.

Please relax. The CT scan has been completed.

MRI 検査

こんにちは．検査伝票をお預かりします．

Hello. May I have your examination slip (form), please?

患者さんには腹部検査の前 3 時間の禁食をお願いしていますが，水分はとっていただいてかまいません．

We ask patients to stop eating 3 hours before the abdominal examination, but they may drink water.

In taking about this test, you should not eat any kind of food three hours before, except water.

服を脱ぐ必要はありませんが，金属製のものは取り除いてください．

> You do not have to take off your clothes, but please remove any metallic objects.

> You do not have to remove your clothes, but please remove any metallic objects.

金属を身に付けていなければ，そのままの格好で検査ができます．

> If you do not wear metals, you can be examined as it is.

金属やアクセサリーを身に付けていると，機械が正常に動作しません．

> The machine will not work properly if you are wearing any metals and accessories.

MRI 検査の方法について説明させてください．

> Let me explain about the methods of MRI examination.

MRI 検査のため少し狭い空間に入っていただきますが，最短時間で実施できるようにします．協力をお願いします．

> You will enter a little small space for MRI examination, but we will try to perform it in the shortest time. Thank you for your cooperation.

(患者) 閉所が苦手な（怖い）のですが．

> I am afraid I don't like small spaces.

> I don't like small places.

I am afraid of enclosed places.

患者 私は閉所恐怖症です．

I am claustrophobic.

> □ 閉所恐怖症　claustrophobia　（〜のおそれ　fear of claustrophobia）

患者 健康には影響しませんか？

Is there any problem with my health?

Does the MRI examination affect my health?

患者 私に副作用はありますか？

Do I have any side effects?

Does it give me any side effects?

注意事項（指示）を守っていただければ，特に問題はありません．

There is no problem if you follow the notes.

If you follow the precautions, there is no problem.

クレジットカードや時計などここに例を挙げたものは，MRI検査室の中には持ち込めませんから注意してください．

Please note that examples such as credit cards and watches cannot be brought into the MRI room.

Credit cards, watches, and other examples cannot be brought into the MRI room.

You cannot bring items like credit cards and watches during the MRI examination.

さもなければ磁気で機能がダメになります．

Otherwise, the magnetic field will ruin their function.

Otherwise, the function will be lost due to magnetism.

Otherwise, the function will be ruined by the magnetism.

ワイヤーの金属は画質にも影響するのでこのガウンに着替えてください．

Please change into this gown because the metal of the wire also affects the imaging quality.

The metal in the wires will affect the image, so please change into this gown.

身体を動かすとうまく検査ができません．動きに弱い検査ですから，なるべく動かないようにお願いします．

If you move your body, we cannot examine well. Since this test is weak to movement, so please do not move as much as possible.

もし気分が悪くなった場合には，このボールを押して（握って）私たちに知らせてください．私たちがすぐに対処します．

If you start to feel discomfort, let us know by squeezing this ball, and we will deal with it right away.

If you feel discomfort, let us know by pressing

this ball. We will deal with it immediately.

痛みや不快なことがありましたら，すぐに私に知らせてくださいね．よろしいですね？

Please let me know immediately if you have any pain or discomfort. OK?

患者〉検査時間はどれくらいかかりますか？

How long does it take for this examination?

How long will the examination take?

How long does the test take?

全部含めてもおおよそ 20 ～ 30 分くらいです．

It takes about 20 to 30 minutes including all.

しかしながら手順により異なります．

But it depends on the procedure.

MRI 検査中に断続的に雑音がしますけれども心配はいりません．

There is intermittent noise during the MRI examination, but do not worry.

Do not worry, there will be intermittent noise during the MRI examination.

雑音が苦手な患者さんには，耳栓やヘッドホンにより緩和させる対策をとっています．

For patients who dislike noise, earplugs and headphones are used to mitigate it.

なるべくこの姿勢を保って，動かないようにお願いします．

Please keep this position as much as possible and do not move.

こちらへどうぞ．この寝台に仰向けで寝て（横たわって）ください．楽にしてください．

This way, please. Please lie on your back on this bed. You can relax.

楽にしてください．MRI 検査は終わりました．

You can now relax. This MRI examination has completed.

Please relax. This MRI examination is over.

The MRI examination has been completed.

患者 どうもありがとう．この後はどうすればいいのですか？

Thank you very much. What should I do after this?

Thank you. What shall I do next now?

MRI のデータをかかりつけ医に持ち帰っていただきますので，受付で少しお待ちください．

Please wait a moment at the reception desk because you will be asked to bring the MRI data to the family doctor.

Please wait at the reception desk for a moment, as you will take the MRI data to your family doctor.

④ 血管造影編

□ 血管造影　angiogram／angiography
□ インターベンショナルラジオロジー　interventional
　radiology（IVR）

検査実施に先立って，患者と家族にインフォームドコンセントを実施してから同意書を取り交わすことが重要です．

> Prior to testing, it is important to obtain informed consent from the patient and their family, and to exchange a consent form.

この血管造影は血管を描出する検査です．

> Angiography is an examination that visualize the blood vessels.

最新の血管造影は DSA（デジタル サブトラクション アンギオグラフィ）で実施されます．

> The latest angiogram (angiography) is carried out in digital subtraction angiography (DSA).

X線撮影を行いながら，カテーテルと呼ばれるチューブを鼠径部から挿入し，標的（頭部／脳／心臓／肺／腹部／骨盤部／四肢）の血管に造影剤を注入します．

> A tube called a catheter is inserted from the groin and inject contrast agent into the target (head / brain / heart / lung / abdominal / pelvic /

limb) blood vessels during X-ray imaging.

さらに，IVR と呼ばれる治療法では，病変近くの動脈に直接薬を注入したり，血管の病変にコイルを詰めたりすることができます．

Furthermore, a method of treatment called IVR can inject medicine directly into the arteries nearby the lesion or set a coil in the lesion of the blood vessel.

IVR は診断と治療を同時に行うことができる血管造影検査です．

IVR is an angiographic examination that allows diagnosis and treatment simultaneously.

IVR は切開手術に比べて患者さんの身体的侵襲度は非常に小さいです．

IVR is much less physical invasion than open surgery for patients.

心臓カテーテル検査においては，バルーンを膨らませて細くなった血管を広げる治療法があります．

There is a technique to widen a narrowed blood vessel with inflated balloon in the case of cardiac catheter exam.

検査時間は，1〜3時間ほどかかります．

It takes about 1 to 3 hours for the examination.

The examination takes about 1 to 3 hours.

検査終了後，病室のベッドで安静にしていただきます．

You should need to rest on the bed in the hospital room after the examination.

After this examination, you should need to rest in the hospital ward.

（患者）**この検査は痛みがあるのですか？**

Do I feel any pain in this test?

Does this examination hurt?

（患者）**この検査ではどのような造影剤を使うのでしょうか？私はアレルギーがありますから．**

What kind of contrast agent will you use for this test? Because I have allergies.

血管造影の検査は造影剤を使用して行います．造影剤はまれに副作用を生じることがあります．あなたはアレルギーや喘息はありませんか？

A contrast medium is utilized in the angiography. It may cause side effects occasionally. Do you have any allergies or asthma?

ヨード剤にアレルギーのある人や妊娠の可能性のある人は検査できませんので，医師にその旨を告げてください．

The patients who are allergic to iodine drugs or who may be pregnant cannot test, so please tell your doctor.

頻度は高くありませんが，ときに検査終了後に吐き気・蕁麻疹・かゆみ・息苦しさなどの副作用が出る場合があります．その際は早めに医師へお申し出ください．

It is not quite often, but sometimes patients experience side effects such as nausea, hives, itches, and stifling. When this happens, please consult the doctor as soon as possible.

- ☐ 吐き気　nausea
- ☐ 蕁麻疹　hives
- ☐ かゆみ　itches
- ☐ 息苦しさ　stifling

（あなたに）モニターを取り付けます．それから，滅菌シーツで覆いますよ．

I will attach the monitor to you. I will cover you with sterile sheets.

検査中に何か変わったことがありましたら，身体を動かさず医師に声をかけてください．

If you feel anything discomfort, please stay still and tell our doctor.

この検査にはによりよい精密な画像を得るために造影剤を使う必要があります.

> This examination needs to use contrast material, so it makes more fine images.

> Using contrast agent is necessary for this examination, so it makes more fine images.

これから造影剤を血管内に入れて検査をしていきます.

> From now, we put the contrast agent in the blood vessel and will examine it.

> We will now start examining your blood vessels. And we use the contrast agent for this examination.

造影剤注入時に多少の灼熱感がありますが,痛みはありません.

> You will feel a slightly hot when the contrast agent is injected, but you feel no pain.

造影剤が注入されたときには少し熱感がありますが体を動かさないでください.

> When the contrast agent is injected, you feel slightly hot, but please stay still.

造影剤が血管の中に入っていくと少しだけ熱くなるような感じがしますが,心配いりません.

> As the contrast agent enters the blood vessels, you feel a little hot, but you do not have to worry.

鼠径部を消毒しますので，少し冷たい感じがします．

When I disinfect your inguinal part, you feel cold.

As I sterilize your inguinal part, you will feel cool.

局所麻酔をしますので，少し痛みます．

You have a little pain when I do local anesthesia.

I am going to apply local anesthesia and this may hurt a little.

これからカテーテルを挿入していきます．

I am going to insert the catheter now.

検査中は動かないでください．

I need you to stay still during the examination.

Please do not move during the examination.

検査後は出血に注意し，安静にしていてください．

Please stay still after the test because you might bleed. So be careful.

You might bleed a little after the test but will be fine if you keep still.

血管撮影検査を始めます．検査時間は 20 分ほどです．

We will begin the angiogram (angiography). It takes about twenty minutes.

We will now start examining your blood vessels. It will take about twenty minutes.

医師の許可が出るまでこのまま右脚を動かさずにいてください.

Please try not to move your right leg until doctor's permission.

Please do not move your right leg until the doctor's permission.

何か必要があれば，ベッドについているボタンで看護師を呼んでください.

If you need assistance, please call the nurse with the button on the bed.

約束を守って，ベッドで静かにしていてください.

Please obey the rules, and stay in your bed.

検査は順調に終了しました.お疲れさまでした.お大事に.

The test was successful. Thank you for your hard work. (You did a good job.)

The examination ended well. Thank you for your good work. (Good job on your work.)

The examination ended well. Thank you so much for your cooperation. You did a great job! Take care.

5 マンモグラフィ編

□ 乳房 X 線検査　mammography
□ 乳房 X 線写真　mammogram

大変長いことお待たせいたしました．（混雑してお待たせした場合）

I am sorry to have kept you waiting so long.

当院では女性の診療放射線技師が乳房撮影を担当しています．

A female radiological technologist is in charge of mammography at our hospital.

彼女がマンモグラフィを実施します．

She carries out the mammography.

マンモグラフィを以前にうけたことがありますか？

Have you ever had a mammography?

乳房撮影をしたことはありますか？

Have you ever had a mammogram?

マンモグラフィ検査について説明します（説明させてください）．

I would like to explain about mammography.

Please let me explain about mammography.

マンモグラフィとは乳房専用の機器（X線検査）のことです.

Mammography is a dedicated device for the breast.

Mammogram is an X-ray examination exclusively for the breast.

マンモグラフィは, 乳房 X 線写真専用の X 線装置で, 乳房を 2 枚の板の間で圧迫して撮影します.

Mammography is a dedicated X-ray machine for mammogram, the breast is photographed by compressing between two plates.

マンモグラフィの放射線が人体へ及ぼす危険性はほとんどありません.

There is almost no risk of radiation from mammography to the human body.

マンモグラフィで受ける放射線の量は約 1〜3 ミリグレイです.

The amount of radiation received by mammogram is about 1 to 3 milligray (mGy).

妊婦さんのおなかの中の胎児に形成異常（奇形）などをきたす放射線量は 100 ミリグレイです.

The radiation dose that causes such as malformation to the fetus in a pregnant woman is 100 milligray (mGy).

☐ 形成異常（奇形）　malformation

乳がんの早期発見のためにもマンモグラフィ検査が有効です.

> Mammography is also effective for early detection of breast cancer.

乳房を圧迫する理由はいくつかあります.

> There are several reasons to compress your breast.

その理由の一つは，乳房を圧迫固定し画像のボケを少なくしてコントラストを良くすることで診断しやすい画像にするためです.

> One of the reasons is to make the image suitable for diagnosis by reducing the blur and improving the contrast, with compression and fixation of the breast.

これは乳房全体を広く描出（視覚化）し，病変を発見しやすくするためです.

> This is because the entire breast is widely visualized and lesions can be easily detected.

乳房を圧迫しながら薄く均等に広げることにより，乳房の中をより鮮明に見ることができます.

> We can see the inside of the breast more clearly by pressing the breast and spreading it thinly and evenly.

上半身の衣服を脱いでください.

> Please take off your clothes from the waist up.
>
> Please remove your clothes from your waist up.

Please take off your upper clothes.

上半身裸になって，ガウンを羽織ってください．

Please be shirtless and put on a hospital gown.

Please remove all your clothing from the waist up and wear a hospital gown.

☐ アクセサリー類をはずしてもらう　remove accessories
☐ 眼鏡をはずしてもらう　take off your glasses
☐ 髪の毛を後ろで縛ってもらう　have your hair tied up behind
☐ 腋の下や胸元をウェットティッシュで拭いてもらう　have your armpit and chest wipe with a wet tissue
☐ 妊娠の可能性の有無を確認　check for possible pregnancy
☐ 豊胸術施行の有無を確認　check for breast implants
☐ ペースメーカーの有無を確認　check if the patient has a pacemaker
☐ シャント術実施の有無を確認　check if shunt operation is performed

ご自分の乳房で特に気になる（押すと痛みやしこりを感じる）部分はどこですか？

Where do you mostly feel the lump when you press your breast?

Where do you mostly feel pain when you pressed your breast?

片側ずつ乳房を圧迫してX線撮影していきます．

We will examine one breast at a time.

We will examine your breast by compressing each one.

One side at a time, the breast is pressed and

X-ray is taken.

圧迫の際に乳房を引っ張ることがあります.

When compressing, I may need to pull on your breast.

もしも我慢ができないようなら言ってください.

If you cannot stand it, please tell me.

Please tell me soon, if you cannot endure it.

痛みや不快なことがありましたら知らせてください.

Please let me know if you have any pain or discomfort.

この黒い平板の上に右（左）の乳房を乗せてください.
（CC；craniocaudal view　頭尾方向撮影）

Please place your right (left) breast on this black plate.

Please put your right (left) breast on this black plate.

右（左）の頬をフェイスガードに付けてください.（CC）

Please put the right (left) cheek on the face guard.

Attach the right (left) cheek to the face guard.

強く圧迫して撮影しますが，我慢できないときにはすぐに声をかけてください．

> I press it strongly and take a mammogram, but if you cannot stand it, tell me immediately.

検査後にはすぐに圧迫板が離れます．板が離れたら，体を楽にしてください．

> The compression plate will be released soon after the examination. When the boards apart, relax your muscles normally.

同じように，もう片方（反対側）の乳房を撮影します．

> We would like to test the opposite breast.
>
> We would like to examine the other breast.

次に，内側から外側へ乳房を圧迫します．
（MLO；mediolateral oblique view　内外斜位方向撮影）

> We will be compressing the breast to extend it from the center of your body.

腋の下を黒い板の角に乗せて体を斜めにしてください．（MLO）

> Please place your armpit on this black plate and tilt your body.

検査終了です．（状況により）

> This examination finished.
>
> The examination is completed / done / over.
>
> The examination has been completed.

画像を確認しますので，ガウンを羽織って椅子に座ってお待ちください．

> Please take on a hospital gown and wait in a chair until I check the image.

> Since I will check the image, please put on a hospital gown and wait in a chair.

マンモグラフィ検診の結果もしも悪性の可能性がある場合，"異常あり，精密検査が必要です" というお知らせがいくことになります．

> If there is a possibility of malignancy as a result of the mammography examination, you will be notified that there is an abnormality and a detailed examination is required.

これは必ずしも乳がんというわけではありませんので，必要以上に心配することはありません．

> This is not necessarily breast cancer, so do not worry too much.

マンモグラフィの検査では悪性の病気だけでなく，良性のものも見つかります．

> Mammography examinations can find benign as well as malignant diseases.

このファイルを持って1階の⑦会計窓口へ行ってください．

> Take this file to the 7 calculation desk on the first floor.

> Please go to number 7 accounting desk on the 1st floor and give them this file.

Useful phrase

Removing your clothes is very important for this examination because it can help us to have a better image of your breast. Do not worry because it is not a dangerous examination. I am here to assist you carefully.

核医学（RI）編

落ち着いて（緊張しないで）くださいね．私がしっかりと補佐いたしますから．

> Please stay calm. I will take good care of you.
>
> I hope I can attend to you carefully and make you feel comfortable.
>
> I am here to assist you, please do not worry.
>
> I will be here to help you every step of the way.

フルネームを確認させていただいてもよろしいですか？

> Could you please confirm your full name?
>
> May I have your full name again?

この部門では微量の放射能をもつ放射性物質を取り扱います．

> We handle a radioactive material having a very small amount of radioactivity in this department.

核医学検査では，放射性同位元素（アイソトープ，RI）と呼ばれる放射線を出す物質を含んだ薬品（放射性医薬品）を注射により体内に投与します．

A drug containing a substance called radioactive isotope (RI) that emit radiation is administered to the body by injection in nuclear tests.

体内に注入する RI からの放射線の量は人体には害がない程度にとても微量です．

The amount of radiation from RI injected into the body is so small that it does not harm the human body.

放射性同位元素には半減期と呼ばれる現象があり，時間の経過とともに放射線を放出する能力（放射能）は半減します．

There is a phenomenon called half-life of radioisotopes, the ability to emit radiation (radioactivity) could be halved over time.

投与後は，装置のベッドで静かに仰向けに寝ている間にガンマカメラという専用のカメラ装置で体内から出てくる放射線を検出します．

After administration, a special device called a gamma camera detects radiation coming out of the body while lie back on the device bed quietly.

ガンマカメラで検出してできた画像をシンチグラフィと呼びます.

The detected image by a gamma camera is called scintigraphy.

この検査は非常に苦痛の少ない検査で,多くの場合,撮像に20〜30分かかります.

This examination is a very painless test, which often takes 20-30 minutes to get image data.

もし助けが必要でしたら,私にお知らせください.お手伝いさせていただきます.

If you need any help, please let me know. I will be glad to help you.

SPECT(単一光子放射コンピュータ断層撮影)検査

SPECT とは,シングル フォトン エミッション CT の略語です.

SPECT is an abbreviation for Single Photon Emission CT.

SPECT は体内に注入した RI(放射性同位元素)の分布状況を断層画像で見る検査のことです.

SPECT is an examination of tomographic images that visualize the distribution of RI (radioactive isotopes) injected into the body.

静脈から RI（放射性同位元素）を注入します．この検査は特に脳血管障害や心疾患の診断で威力を発揮します．

The RI (radioisotope) is injected from the vein of patient. This examination is particularly effective in the diagnosis of cerebrovascular disorders and heart diseases.

SPECT では従来の CT では表わすことができなかった血流量や代謝機能の情報が得られます．

SPECT provides information on blood flow and metabolic function that cannot be expressed by conventional CT scan.

血流状態がよくわかり，血液が流れていない虚血領域を確認することができます．

This allows us to better understand the blood flow condition and check the ischemic area where blood is not flowing.

Blood flow conditions can be understood well, and the ischemic area where blood is not flowing can be confirmed.

- ☐ 血流　blood flow
- ☐ 虚血領域　ischemic area

これにより初期の脳梗塞やその他の脳血管障害，一過性脳虚血発作，回復可能な脳卒中，てんかん，アルツハイマー病，パーキンソン病，脳腫瘍などが診断できます．

This can diagnose early cerebral infarction and other cerebrovascular disorders, transient ischemic attack, fully resilient stroke, epilepsy,

Alzheimer's disease, Parkinson's disease, and brain tumors.

☐ 脳梗塞　cerebral infarction
☐ 脳血管障害　cerebrovascular disorder
☐ 一過性脳虚血発作　transient ischemic attack
☐ 脳卒中　stroke
☐ てんかん　epilepsy
☐ アルツハイマー病　Alzheimer's disease
☐ パーキンソン病　Parkinson's disease
☐ 脳腫瘍　brain tumor

PET-CT 検査

PET-CT 検査は生体の生理機能や代謝機能を診断できます.

PET-CT tests can diagnose the physiological and metabolic functions of living body.

PET-CT 検査はてんかんや虚血性心疾患および悪性腫瘍の診断に用いられます.

PET-CT tests are used to diagnose epilepsy, ischemic heart disease, and malignant tumors.

☐ 虚血性心疾患　ischemic heart disease

PET-CT 検査では全身のがんのスクリーニングが可能です.

PET-CT examination (test) allow screening for cancer throughout the body.

PET-CT 装置はがんの早期発見に有効です.

The PET-CT device is effective for early

detection of cancer.

PET-CT では他の画像診断では見つからない小さながんの発見が可能です.

> PET-CT can detect small cancers that cannot be found with other diagnostic imaging.

PET 検査前 (と検査中) には目を使わないように安静にする必要があります.

> You need to take a rest so as not to use your eyes before the PET test.

> You have to take a rest and close your eyes before and during the test.

これから FDG という薬品を使います.

> I am going to use a drug called FDG.

検査終了後には私が声をかけるまで安静にしていてください.

> Please rest until I speak to you after the examination.

> Please take a rest until I talk to you after the examination.

アイソトープ検査

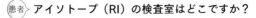患者 **アイソトープ (RI) の検査室はどこですか？**

> Where is the radioisotope (RI) division?

Could you tell me where the RI room is?

I wonder if you could tell me where the nuclear medicine department is?

はい，ここがそうです．ご用件は何でしょうか？

Yes, it is here. What can I do for you?

Yes, that is right. How may I help you? (How can I help you?)

RI の予約票をお預かりいたします（受け取ります）．

I will receive your RI booking slip.

I will receive your RI reservation form.

この黄色いスリッパに履き替えて中にお入りください．

Please put on these yellow slippers and come inside.

Please change to these yellow slippers from your shoes and enter.

 これ（RI）は何のための検査ですか？

What is this RI test for?

What kind of examination is this RI test?

Please tell me about this RI examination.

今回の検査は腎機能*の検査です．

We are going to examine your kidney function.

トレーサ（アイソトープの薬）を静脈注射して，ガンマカメラという装置で撮影をします．

> We are going to inject a tracer into your vein and to take imaging data (pictures) using a device called a "gamma camera."

□ トレーサ　tracer（ガンマ線を放出する放射性合成物や放射性薬品）

(患者) この RI 検査にはどのくらい時間がかかりますか？

> How long does it take for this RI examination?
> How long does the RI examination take?

検査に約 30 分（1 時間）かかります．

> It will take about 30 minutes (1 hour).

今から医師があなたに RI の注射をします．そして 3 時間後から撮像します．

> From now, the doctor will give you an RI injection. And we take your images from 3 hours later.

注射後，トレーサが目的部位に行き渡るまでに時間がかかるのです．

> It takes time for the tracer to reach the area we

want to examine after injection.

あなたの RI 検査は 15：30 から撮像が開始されます．

Your RI imaging starts from 15:30.

検査が終わったら何か食べてもいいですよ．

You can have something to eat after the examination.

You may eat something after the examination.

検査が終わるまで食事はとらないでください（禁食してください）．

Please do not eat until the test is over.

Please do not eat anything until this test is done.

Please continue to fast until after the examination.

You are not allowed to eat anything until the test is done.

検査を優先して朝食は食べないようにしてください．

Do not eat breakfast in order to prioritize this test.

Please do not eat the breakfast in order to give priority to this examination.

昼食は検査が終わるまで食べないでください．

Please do not eat lunch until after the examination.

Please do not eat lunch until the examination is done.

核医学（RI）編

お茶やお水でしたら，多少飲んでもかまいません．

If it is tea or water, you can drink some.

You can have a little tea or water.

食事制限は検査部位や使用薬剤によって異なります．

Dietary restrictions vary depending on the test part and the drug used for the test.

この検査はヨウ素のコントロールが必要なため，検査前1週間は海藻類・貝類を食べないでください．

For this examination, you need to control the amount of iodine in your body, therefore please do not eat seaweeds and shellfishes during one week before the examination.

検査の前処置として，飲み薬や下剤などが処方される場合があります．

As a pretreatment for the test, you may be prescribed medicine or laxatives.

検査自体は痛くも苦しくもありません．アイソトープの薬を注射するときに医師が注射針を刺すので多少の痛みがあります．

The examination itself is not painful, but you will feel the pain of injecting RI slightly.

The test itself is neither painful nor difficult. But there is some pain (to you) because the doctor inserts a needle when injecting the isotope medicine.

心電図をとりますので，上半身裸になってこの検査着に着替えてください．

> We are going to take an electrocardiogram (ECG, EKG), so please take off your clothes from the waist up and put on this gown.

脳波もとります．

> We will also take your EEG (electroencephalogram).

> You will undergo EEG (electroencephalogram).

金属のついている服や下着を脱いでください．金属類はこの検査の妨げになります．

> Please remove any items of clothing that have any kind of metal. Metals disturb this examination.

着替え終わったら，検査の前に（トイレに行って）排尿してください．

> Please go to the restroom and urinate before the examination if you finish changing your clothes.

> Before the examination, you need to urinate first if you finish changing your clothes.

良好な画像を得るため，まず膀胱を空にしておく必要があるのです．

> To have a better imaging, you need to empty your bladder first.

入れ歯，ヘアピン，ネックレスその他の装身具，眼鏡，補聴器などを外してください．かごの中に全部入れてください．

Please remove your false teeth, hairpins, necklaces and any other accessories, eyeglasses, hearing aid, and so on. And put them in this basket.

□ ヘアピン　hairpin
□ ネックレス　necklace
□ 装身具　accessory／ornament
□ 眼鏡　eyeglasses／spectacles
□ 補聴器　hearing aid／otophone

患者 この服は着たままでいいですか？

I am wearing these clothes, and is it all right?

服は大丈夫です．でもその金属類だけは外してください．

It is all right. But please take off only metals.

この台の上に仰向けに寝てください．

Lie on your back on this examination table, please.

両腕を上に挙げてください．

Please raise both your arms up.

両目を閉じてください．私があなたを迎えに来るまで安静にしていてください．

Close (both of) your eyes. Please rest quietly in bed until I come to pick you up.

良好な画像を得るために，目を使わないよう目隠しをします．

> In order to get the best images, I am going to cover your eyes with this blindfold not to use your eyes.

> In order to get the best images, it does help if we cover your eyes with this blindfold.

このままの状態で5分ほど動かないでください．

> Please do not move. Please keep the same condition about five minutes.

> Please stay still for approximately five minutes.

右腕に注射します．袖をまくり上げてください．

> We are going to give you an injection in your right arm. Please roll up your sleeve.

両手は体の脇に置いてください．お腹の上に乗せないようご注意ください．

> Put your hands on the side of your body. Please make sure not to rest them on your abdomen.

> Put your hands on the side of your body and please be careful not to put them on your abdomen.

何かあったときには，動かないで私たちを呼んでください．

> Please stay still. Tell us if you feel any discomfort.

> When something happens, please try not to move and tell us.

迎えにきますので，ここで待っていてください．

I will come to pick you up, so please wait here.

検査は無事に終了しました．お疲れさまでした．

This RI examination has been completed. You did a good job.

お大事になさってください．

Please take care of yourself.

Take good care.

早く回復なさってください．

I hope you will be better soon.

I wish you a fast recovery.

ラジオアイソトープの画像
☐ 機能画像　functional image
☐ 代謝画像　metabolism image
☐ 形態画像　morphological image

放射線治療編

□ 放射線治療部門　radiation therapy department／
radiotherapy department

放射線治療では，患者さんへしっかりと説明した後に，患者さんの理解を得て治療への協力を得ることが重要です．これがいわゆるインフォームドコンセント（IC）です．

> It is important in radiation therapy to get the patient's understanding and cooperation in treatment after giving a thorough explanation to the patient. This is the so-called informed consent (IC).

患者 > 放射線治療部門はどこか教えてください？

> Where is the radiation therapy department?
>
> How can I arrive the radiation therapy department?
>
> Could you tell me where the radiotherapy department is?
>
> I wonder if you could tell me where the radiotherapy department is?

どうかなさいましたか？／お手伝いいたしましょうか？／お困りですか？

> What can I do for you?

—77—

How may I help you?

What are your symptoms?

How are you feeling?

この放射線治療の期間は約4週間です．

The radiation therapy probably takes 4 weeks.

It takes about 4 weeks for this radiation therapy.

これから約1ヵ月間，私と一緒に放射線治療をがんばって受けてくださいね．

Please do your best to undergo radiation therapy with me for about a month from now.

あなたのために精一杯がんばります．／しっかり支援いたします．

I am here for you.

I am here to assist you.

I will do my best to assist you.

I will take good care of you.

あなたに早くよくなって（元気になって）もらいたいです．

I wish you a fast recovery.

I hope you will be better soon.

リニアックと呼ばれる装置を使って患者さんに放射線治療を行います．

Radiation therapy is performed on the patient using a device called LINAC (linear accelerator).

I give radiation therapy to a patient using a device named linear accelerator.

 患者 大丈夫でしょうか？ いまだ放射線がこわいのですが.

Will it be all right? I'm worried about the radiation yet. (I'm afraid of the radiation yet.)

放射線治療に使用される放射線の量はX線検査よりかなり多いですが，悪い病気を治すための治療ですから，ご理解とご協力をお願いします.

The dose for radiation therapy is quite more than X-ray test, but I would like your understanding and cooperation because it is treatment to cure a bad disease.

健常組織にダメージを与えないように，がん組織に集中して局部的に治療をします.

Local treatment is usually focused on cancer tissue so as not to damage healthy tissue.

Local treatment is usually focused on cancer tissue, this is done not to damage healthy tissue.

 患者 放射線治療がつらくなったら途中でやめてもよいのですか？

Can I stop the radiation therapy when it becomes uncomfortable for me?

Can I discontinue this therapy when I feel sick?

途中で治療をやめると腫瘍（がん）が増悪する場合があるためそうしないほうがよいと思います．

> I do not hope you will give up the treatment halfway because that may cause exacerbation of the tumor.

> I do not advise you to stop the treatment halfway because that will speed up the spread of the cancer cells.

この治療について言っておくと，少しつらさを感じて途中で治療を中止したくなるかもしれませんが，がん細胞の増殖を早めてしまうことがあるので，治療の中止は勧められません．

> I have to warn you about this treatment, you might experience some discomfort and think of giving up the treatment while in progress, but I advise you not to discontinue the treatment because spread of the cancer cells may accelerate.

（放射線治療では）まず最初に患者さんのシミュレーションをします．

> We simulate the patient first.

> First, we do simulation of the patient.

> I will simulate the patient of radiotherapy first.

> I will do the patient simulation first.

> First of all, we do the patient simulation.

> For the radiotherapy, first we will simulate the patient.

シミュレーションというのは患者さんごとの治療計画を意味する準備行為です.

> Simulation is the preparatory action meaning the treatment plan of each patient.

シミュレーションでは，治療計画用の CT 検査で患者さんの病巣を定めます.

> In the simulation, the patient's lesion is determined by CT examination for the treatment plan.

シミュレーションの際（後）に，治療用の固定具をつけます.

> During the simulation, I will put the therapeutic fixture for you.

> In the case of simulation, I will put the therapeutic fixture for you.

> After the simulation, I will put the therapeutic fixture for you.

シミュレーションの際（後）に，皮膚の表面に印をつけます.

> During the simulation, I will mark the surface of the skin.

> In the case of simulation, I will mark the surface of the skin.

> After the simulation, I will mark the surface of the skin.

シミュレーション後，皮膚の表面に印を付け，治療用の固定具を着けます.

> After the simulation, I will mark the surface of

your skin and put the therapeutic fixture for you.

体表に印をつけますが，皮膚インキという特別な液を使います．

I will mark the surface of your body and use the special liquid named the dermatologic ink.

体の表面に印を付けさせてください．なるべく消えないように注意なさってください．

Let me mark the surface of your body. Please be careful not to disappear as much as possible.

Keep the surface of the body be marked. Please be careful not to disappear as much as possible.

放射線治療を受けている期間中はあなたの体のマークした線が消えないように注意しましょう．

Be careful not to erase the marked lines on your body while you are undergoing radiation therapy.

激しい運動をすると汗でマークした線が消えてしまう可能性が高くなりますので，放射線治療期間中は避けていただくようお願いします．

It is highly possible that the marked line will disappear due to sweat in heavy exercise, so please avoid it during the radiotherapy period.

Useful phrase

Please let me mark the surface of your body and please be careful not to disappear the mark as much as possible.

それは痛いですか？　怖いのです.

Is it painful? I'm afraid of it.

Does it hurt? I'm scared of it.

大丈夫です，痛くはないですよ.

All right, you do not have a pain.

It is okay, you will not be hurt.

放射線治療のために入院する必要がありますか？

Must I be hospitalized for radiation therapy?

Do I have to be hospitalized for radiation therapy?

仕事（通常の生活）を続けられるので外来の患者さんが多いです.

There are a lot of outpatients because it is possible to continue their works.

There are a lot of outpatients because it is possible to continue normal life.

放射線による影響で皮膚炎が出やすい患者さんもいますので,温泉入浴などについては医療スタッフにご相談ください.

Some patients are prone to dermatitis due to radiation, so please consult your medical staff about bathing in hot springs.

放射線治療期間中は，連日の来院と放射線照射により体が疲れやすくなります.

During the radiotherapy period, your body may

放射線治療編

get tired easily due to daily visits and irradiation.

栄養のあるバランスのとれた食事と充分な睡眠を心がけてください.

Please keep a nutritious, balanced diet, and good sleep.

(患者) 放射線治療の予定（日程）を教えてください.

Please tell me the schedule of the radiation therapy.

患者さんには月曜日から金曜日まで（平日に）放射線治療をしますので土曜日と日曜日（週末）は休息をとってください.

We do radiation therapy to patients from Monday through Friday, and please [take a] rest on Saturday and Sunday.

Patients should undergo radiation therapy only on weekdays and must take a rest on weekends.

月曜日から金曜日まで週5日，分割照射という放射線治療を行います.

We will conduct radiation therapy called fractionated irradiation five days a week from Monday to Friday.

From Monday to Friday, radiation therapy is performed five days a week as fractionated irradiation.

これは分割照射法といって，何回かに分けて少しずつ病巣に放射線を集中させます．

This is called a fractionated irradiation method, and radiation is gradually concentrated to the lesion by dividing into several times.

We call the method "fractionated irradiation" that centralize radiation little by little to the lesion.

照射位置の確認を定期的に行い，週1回，医師の診察を受けます．

The irradiation position is checked regularly, and you see a doctor once a week.

血液のがんの治療では全身照射（TBI）という治療方法があります．

There is a method called total body irradiation (TBI) for the treatment of blood cancer.

白血病などの血液のがんの治療では全身照射を行います．

Total body irradiation (TBI) is used for treatment of blood cancers such as leukemia.

この全身照射は造血幹細胞移植の前処置です．

This total body irradiation is a pretreatment for hematopoietic stem cell transplantation.

患者 この放射線治療には副作用がありますか？

Does this radiation therapy have any side effects on me?

放射線治療編

Does this radiotherapy cause me side effects?

（患者）放射線治療を受けた後に悪影響がありますか？

Are there any bad effects after I have this radiation therapy?

放射線治療には，根治・姑息・術前・術中・術後照射があります．

Radiation therapy includes curative, makeshift, preoperative, intraoperative, and postoperative irradiation.

治療室での放射線治療において，正確な位置に照射を行います．

We irradiate the correct position in radiotherapy in the treatment room.

急性期の副作用は治療中や治療直後に起きる可能性があるものです．

Side effects of acute phase can occur during or immediately after treatment.

Side effects in the acute stage can occur during or immediately after treatment.

急性期の副作用として，全身的なものでは食欲不振や貧血，局所的なものでは脱毛や紅斑などがあります．

Side effects of acute phase include loss of appetite and anemia as systemic ones, hair loss and erythema as local ones.

晩発期になってから副作用が発生する場合もあります.

Side effects may occur in the later phase.

Side effects may sometimes happen in the later phase.

髪の毛が抜けたりしますが,放射線治療の終了後にはまた生えてきますよ.

Your hair will fall out, but after the radiation treatment, your hair will grow again.

Hair falls out, but after the radiation therapy, the hair grows again.

この治療時間は5分程度です.

This treatment time takes about five minutes.

It takes about five minutes for this therapy.

それではこれから放射線治療を開始します.このままの姿勢を保っていてください.

Then I will start radiation therapy from now. Please stay still in the same position.

We will now start the radiation therapy. Please try not to move. (Please do not move.)

何か助けが必要になったらすぐに私に知らせてください.喜んで力になりますよ.

If you need any help, please let me know immediately. I will be glad to help you.

何か変わったことがあったら，大きな声を出してください．
そのときは私が治療を中断して中に入ってきます．

> If anything unusual happens, please talk loudly.
> Then I will interrupt the treatment and come in.

> If there is any problem, please talk loudly. I will
> interrupt the treatment and come in to attend to
> you.

8 受付・案内編

受　付

□ 受付　reception desk

お手伝いいたしましょうか？／何かご用でしょうか？

Can I help you?

How can I help you?

May I help you?

Can I help you with anything?

What can I do for you? 丁寧 / 推奨

How may I help you? 丁寧 / 推奨

何かお困りでしょうか？

Is something bothering you?

Do you have any trouble?

What seems to be the problem?

何をお探しですか？

What are you looking for?

Are you looking for something?

受付・案内編

何とおっしゃいましたか？／もう一度（ゆっくり）話していただけますか？（聞き直す場合）

What did you say?

I beg your pardon?

Pardon me. Would you say that again, please?

Excuse me. Could you repeat that, please?

I am sorry. Can you speak more slowly, please?

今日は何の検査を受けに来られましたか？

What examination would you undergo today?

What kind of examination do you need today?

医療保険証をお持ちですか？

Do you have a medical insurance card?

この検査を受けるには予約が必要です．

Reservations are required to take this medical test.

You will need a reservation to take the medical examination.

今日受ける検査の予約はしていますか？

Did you make a reservation for today's examination?

Do you have an appointment today?

その検査の予約は主治医を通して行います．

A reservation for the test will be made through

your attending physician.

Your attending physician will reserve the examination.

☐ 主治医　attending physician

主治医に検査の内容を確認しますので，椅子に座ってお待ちください．

Please take a seat until I confirm the examination to the attending physician.

Please sit in a chair and wait until I check the contents of the examination with your doctor.

あなたは主治（担当）医の名前を知っていますか？

Do you know your attending physician's name?

Do you know the name of your attending physician?

あなたはかかりつけ医の名前を知っていますか？（名前を教えてください.）

Do you know your family doctor's name?

Please tell me who your family doctor is.

Please tell me the name of your family doctor.

☐ かかりつけ医　family doctor

誰から放射線科に行くように言われましたか？

Who told you to go to the radiology department?

あなたは主治医から何科に行くように言われましたか？

Which department were you directed to go to from your attending doctor?

Please tell me where the department indicated by your attending doctor is?

何の検査に行くように言われましたか？

What test were you indicated to go for?

What kind of examination were you indicated to take?

☐ 検査を受ける　be examined／go through examination／undergo an examination

何という名前の病院から来ましたか？

Which hospital did you come from?

I wonder if you could tell me the name of the hospital you attended.

今日受ける検査の予約をしていますか？

Did you make the reservation for today's medical examination?

☐ 検査の予約票　reservation form／booking slip

混雑しているので，予約の時間には検査が開始できません．

We cannot start the medical examination on time because of congestion.

As it is crowded, the examination cannot start at

the time of the reservation.

救急患者が来るので，検査の開始が5分ほど遅れてしまいそうです．

The examination will start about 5 minutes later due to an emergency patient arriving.

As an emergency patient will come, the start of the examination seems to be late approximately five minutes.

検査の内容や患者様の状態により，検査の順番が前後することがあります．

The order of examination may alter depending on the exam contents and the condition of the patients.

By the contents of the examination and the state of patients, a turn of the examination may be mixed up.

検査の結果が出るまで1時間ほどかかります．

It will take about an hour for the results to arrive.

It takes approximately 1 hour until a result of the examination is given.

A result of the examination takes approximately 1 hour until it appears.

検査の結果が出ましたら，レポートと画像データをここでお渡しします．

I will give your reports and image data to you

after the results are arrived.

When the result of your examination comes out, I bring the report and image data here.

検査結果が出ましたらお名前をお呼びします．

We will call your name when the results arrived.

名前を呼ばれるまで椅子に座って待っていてください．

Please take a seat until your name is called.

Please have a seat and wait until your name is called.

名前を呼んでもいらっしゃらないときには，ここで検査結果を保管しておきます．

If you are not there when your name is called, we will retain your results here.

If you are not there when I call your name, I keep the test result here.

いつ（何曜日）に検査結果を取りに来ますか？

When will you come and receive your test result?

What day of the week will you come here for your result?

When (What day) will you arrive to take your test results?

この受付は朝8時30分から夕方5時まで開いています．

The reception is open from eight thirty in the morning to five in the afternoon (evening).

This reception opens at 8:30 a.m. until 5:00 p.m.

検査結果は明日東京病院に FAX しますので，明日以降，東京病院に行ってください．

> We will fax the results to Tokyo Hospital tomorrow. Please go to Tokyo Hospital after tomorrow.

> As the test result will be faxed to Tokyo Hospital tomorrow, please go to the Tokyo Hospital after tomorrow.

検査結果はこちらから東京病院に郵送します．

> We will mail your test result to Tokyo Hospital.

> Your test result will be mailed from this hospital to Tokyo Hospital.

検査の結果は紹介元の病院（診療所）の医師へ郵送します．

> The result of the examination will be sent to your hospital (medical office) doctor.

検査結果はこちらから主治医に郵送します．5日後に診察に行ってください．

> We will mail the results to your physician. Please get a consultation 5 days later.

> We will mail test result to your attending physician. Please go for a medical consultation after 5 days.

今回の検査の結果は主治医（かかりつけ医）が説明します．
ここでは検査結果の説明はしません．

> The results will be explained to you by your attending physician (family doctor), so I do not tell about the results here.

> The attending physician (family doctor) explains the result of this examination. I do not explain the test result here.

かかりつけの医師に今日の結果をお聞きください．

> Please ask your family doctor about today's test result.

次回診察時にかかりつけの医師から結果をお聞きください．

> Please ask your family doctor about the result at your next consultation.

> Ask your family doctor about the result at the next consultation.

次はいつ東京病院（診療所）に行く予定ですか？

> When should you go to Tokyo Hospital (medical office) next time?

> When are you going to go to the Tokyo Hospital (medical office) next time?

今度いつ東京病院（診療所）に行くように医師から言われていますか？

> When is the date recommended by the doctor to go to the Tokyo Hospital (medical office) next time?

Could you tell me the designated day to go to the Tokyo Hospital (medical office) next time?

次は２階の臨床検査の受付へ行ってください（お越しください）.

Then, please go to clinical laboratory reception on the 2nd floor.

Next, please come to clinical laboratory reception on the second floor.

次は４階の採血室受付へ行ってください（お越しください）.

Then, please go to blood sampling reception on the 4th floor.

Next, please come to the blood sampling room on the fourth floor.

放射線科の受付前のエレベータをお使いください.

Please take the elevator in front of radiology reception.

Please use the elevator in front of the radiology reception desk.

放射線科受付前のエレベータで７階へ上がってください.

Please go to the 7th floor by using the elevator in front of radiology reception.

Please go up to the seventh floor by the elevator in front of the radiology reception desk.

右斜め前の受付へファイルを出してください．

Please give the file to reception desk diagonally forward right.

Please give the file to reception located diagonally forward right.

外来診察室へお戻りください．

Please go back to the consultation room of the outpatient.

Please come back to the consulting room of the outpatient department.

1階救急外来へ戻ってこのファイルをお出しください．

Please go back to the emergency room and give this file to the staff.

Please go back to the first aid department, and hand over the file.

正面玄関ロビーにある計算受付に行って，このファイルを渡してください．そして，会計（支払い）をしてください．

Please go to the front reception and hand them this file. Make all payments there, please.

すべての手続き（検査など）を済ませてからご自宅へお帰りください．

Please return to your home after finishing all your procedure.

他にご質問はありますか？

Do you have any questions?

Are there any questions?

気分が悪くありませんか？

Do you feel sick?

Do you feel any discomfort?

ありがとうございます．

Thanks a lot.

Thanks for your help.

Thank you very much.

I appreciate your cooperation.

どういたしまして．

You are welcome.

Do not mention it.

Not at all.

No problem.

Sure.

お大事になさってください．

I wish you a fast recovery.

We hope you feel better soon.

Please take care of yourself.

Please take care.

受付・案内編

外来・入院案内

○○大学病院は，厚生労働省認定の特別機能病院で，高度な医療を提供しています.

○○ University Hospital is a "Special Functioning Hospital" certified by the Ministry of Health, Labor and Welfare, which provides high-level, advanced medical care.

初めて○○大学病院を訪れる海外からの患者さんで，日本の公的健康保険に加入していない方は，予約クリニックまたはセカンドオピニオンサービスの受診をおすすめします.

International patients without Japanese public health insurance visiting ○○ University Hospital for the first time are welcome to be seen at our Reservation Clinic or Second Opinion Service.

予約クリニックでは，待ち時間がほとんどまたはまったくなく，選ばれた医師たちが高度な医療を提供しています.

In the Reservation Clinic, a select group of physicians provide high-level medical care with little or no waiting time.

この診療科は検査に十分な時間を確保しながら安全で高度な医療を確保するために，予約制でのみ提供されています.

This clinical department is offered by appointment only in order to ensure safe, advanced medical care while allowing for sufficient time for examination.

日本に短期滞在で緊急の治療が必要な場合は，国際医療部門に相談してください．

> If you are in Japan for a short stay and require urgent medical treatment, please contact the Department of International Healthcare for a consultation.

病院を訪れるときには身分証明書としてパスポートを必ず持参してください．

> When visiting the hospital be sure to bring your passport for personal identification.

日本の居住者はパスポートの所持や提示は必要ありません．代わりに，在留資格証と日本の公的医療保険証をご持参ください．

> Residents of Japan are not required to carry or present their passports. Instead, please bring your residence identification card and your Japanese public healthcare insurance card if available.

ご予約当日は，まず○○大学病院の国際医療科へ寄っていただき，B棟3階の予約クリニックに行ってください．身分証明書としてパスポートを持参してください．

> On the day of your appointment, please stop first at the ○○ University Hospital Department of International Healthcare, and then go to the Reservation Clinic on the 3rd floor of Building B. Make sure to bring your passport for personal identification.

受付・案内編

アンケートの記入も必要ですので，予約時間の 30 分前にお越しください．詳細については，医療コーディネータにお問い合わせください

> You will also need to fill out a questionnaire, so please come 30 minutes before your appointment time. For more detailed information, inquire with your medical coordinator.

相談にお越しの際は，より安全で信頼性の高い医療を提供するために，以前診察を受けた医療機関から患者紹介書類（紹介状）をお持ちください．

> To provide safer and more reliable medical care, we ask that you bring a patient referral document (letter of referral) from the medical institution where you were previously seen when you come for your consultation.

すでに日本の病院や診療所からの紹介状を持っている人は，母国からの診断書や検査結果は必要ありません．

> People who already have a letter of referral from a hospital or clinic in Japan do not need a medical certificate or test results from their home country.

紹介状をお持ちでない場合は，5,500 円（税込）の追加初期費用が課金されます．

> If you do not have a referral letter, you will be charged an additional initial fee of 5,500 yen (tax included).

かかりつけ医からの紹介状をご提出ください.

Please submit the referral letter here from your family doctor.

事前に医師に直接予約をした場合を除き,紹介状で指名された医師に診てもらうことはできません.その日の初診を担当する医師が診察します.

Unless you have made an appointment directly with the doctor in advance, you may not be able to see the doctor to whom your letter of referral is specifically addressed. You will be seen by the doctor who is in charge of first visits on that day.

病院にお越しになる際には,パスポート,母国や日本の診療所からの診療要約や検査結果など,できるだけ多くの医療情報を持参してください.

When you come to the hospital, please bring your passport, and as much medical information as you can from your home country or from local clinics of Japan, such as medical summaries or test results.

デジタル画像をお持ちの方は,CD-ROM(DICOM 形式)をご持参ください.

If you have digital images, please bring a CD-ROM (DICOM format).

受付・案内編

外国の病院から○○大学病院に **CD-ROM** でデジタル画像を提出する場合は，DICOM 形式で保存してください．

If you are submitting digital images on a CD-ROM from a foreign hospital to ○○ University Hospital, be sure to save them in the DICOM format.

他の形式のデータは私たちのシステムにアップロードすることはできません．

Data in other formats cannot be uploaded into our system.

日本語を話さない患者さんは医療通訳者と一緒に病院にお越しください．

Patients who do not speak Japanese should always come to the hospital together with a medical interpreter.

医療通訳者が同伴しない方は当日診察できない場合がありますのでご注意ください．

Please notice that people without a medical interpreter may not be able to see a doctor on that day.

医療通訳者が同伴しない場合は，国際診療部門に電話して，一般内科の英語を話す医師との初診について話し合ってください．

If you are unable to come with an interpreter, please call the International Department to discuss an initial consultation with an English-speaking doctor in the Department of General

Internal Medicine.

病院に提出する書類は日本語か英語に翻訳してください．

Please translate all documents to be submitted to the hospital into Japanese or English.

患者さんは医療通訳者のみお連れになってください．

We ask that patients come only with a medical interpreter.

家族や友人が同行したい場合は，お一人だけお連れください．

If a family member or friend would like to accompany you, please bring only one person.

外来診療所では，病気や状態によっては同日の検査ができない場合があります．

In the outpatient clinics, there may be times when an examination on the same day is not possible depending on the disease or condition.

一般診療部門は月曜日から金曜日の午前 8 時 30 分から午後 3 時までの診療時間中に患者さんを受け入れます．

The General Medicine Clinic accepts patients during clinic business hours from 8:30 am to 3 pm, Monday through Friday.

受付・案内編

受付時間は病院の部署によって異なる場合があります．

Reception hours may differ depending on the hospital department.

ご来院予定の診療部門のホームページをご確認ください.

Please check the website page of the department you plan to visit.

この病院では平日の午後1時から午後3時までが面会時間と決まっています.

Visiting hours are determined from 1 pm to 3 pm on weekdays at this hospital.

予約クリニックの受付で処方された薬の受け取り,支払いが可能です.

You can receive prescribed medication and make payments at the Reservation Clinic reception desk.

支払いは現金または以下のクレジットカードで行うことができます.

Payment can be made in cash or using the following credit cards.

病院にお越しの際は,可能な限り公共交通機関をご利用ください.

Please use public transportation whenever possible when coming to the hospital.

外来の階はすべて,飲食は禁止されています.

Eating and drinking are prohibited on all outpatient floors.

１号館１階のレストラン，病院メインエントランスの喫茶店，Ｃ棟１階とＢ棟１階のコンビニエンスストアがあります．

Food and drink are available in the restaurant on the 1st floor of Building 1, coffee shop (cafe) at the hospital main entrance, and convenience stores located both on the ground floor of Building C and the 1st floor of Building B.

携帯電話をサイレントモードに設定し，指定エリア（電話エリア）以外の電話での通話はご遠慮ください．

Please set mobile phones to silent mode, and refrain from talking on the phone except in designated areas (phone areas).

病院敷地内や周辺地域での喫煙は禁止されています．

Smoking is prohibited anywhere on the hospital grounds and in surrounding areas.

病院敷地内での写真とビデオの撮影は禁止されています．

Photos and video are prohibited anywhere on the hospital grounds.

ご理解・ご協力をお願いいたします．

We ask for your understanding and cooperation.

ご不便をおかけして申し訳ございませんが，ご理解とご協力をお願いいたします．

We apologize for the inconvenience and appreciate your understanding and cooperation.

心配でしたらお電話ください.

Call us if you are worried.

ご不明な点がありましたらお電話ください.

Please call us if you have any concerns.

疑問点がありましたら，すぐに私にお尋ねください.

If you notice anything doubtful, please ask me immediately.

急なご病気を聞きお見舞い申し上げます.

I would like to express my sympathy on your sudden illness.

「患者が健康に生きること」こそが私たちの望みです.

"Patients live healthy" is our hope.

$\mathsf{T_{ER}M_S}$ 用語集

身体部位・組織・姿勢

仰向け（に横になってください）
       (Lie) on your back／face up

顎	chin
足首	ankle
足趾 あしゅび（つまさき）	
	toe
胃	stomach
位置／位置決め	position／positioning
咽喉（のど）	throat
うつぶせ	on your stomach／face down
腋窩（脇の下）	axilla／armpit
横行結腸	transverse colon
顔	face
（下）顎	chin
額（ひたい）	forehead
下行結腸	descending colon
肩	shoulder
肝臓	liver
冠動脈	coronary artery
気管	trachea
気管支	bronchi
胸郭	rib cage
胸部	chest
頸椎	cervical vertebrae（spine）
頸動脈	carotid artery
脛部（脛 すね）	shin

KUB（腎臓・尿管・膀胱）

	kidney, ureter, and bladder
血液	blood
血管	blood vessel
甲状腺	thyroid gland
肛門	anus
股関節	hip joint
腰	waist
骨盤	pelvis
三尖弁	tricuspid valve
四肢（手足）	limbs
姿勢	position（positioning）
十二指腸	duodenum
上顎	jaw
上行結腸	ascending colon
小腸	small intestine
静脈	vein
食道	esophagus
心臓	heart
腎臓	kidney
膵臓	pancreas
生殖器	genitals
背骨／背中	spine／back
前立腺	prostate
僧帽弁	mitral valve
鼠径部	groin／inguinal region
組織	tissue
大腿（太もも）	thigh
大腿動脈	femoral artery

大腸	large intestine
大動脈	aorta
大動脈弁	aortic valve
胆嚢	gallbladder
腸壁	intestinal wall
直腸	rectum
殿部（尻）	buttocks
頭部	head
動脈	artery
軟部組織	soft tissue
乳腺	mammary gland
乳房	breast
尿管	ureter
粘膜	mucous membrane／mucosa
脳	brain
肺	lungs
肺動脈	pulmonary artery
肺動脈弁	pulmonary（artery）valve
脾臓	spleen
腹部	abdomen
ふくらはぎ（腓腸）	calf
分泌腺	secretory gland
膀胱	bladder
頬	cheek
胸	chest
眼	eyes
目的部位	target area
（輸）尿管	ureter
腰椎	lumbar vertebra（vertebrae）

用語集

肋骨	rib

症状・病名・身体の機能

悪性腫瘍	malignant tumor
あざ／打撲傷	bruise
足白癬（水虫）	tinea pedis／athlete's foot
アテローム	atheroma
アメーバ赤痢	amebic dysentery
アルツハイマー病	Alzheimer's disease
アレルギー	allergy
胃潰瘍	gastric ulcer
息切れ	shortness of breath
息苦しさ	stifling
意識喪失	unconsciousness
痛み／痛い	pain／ache／sore
胃腸炎	gastroenteritis
胃腸疾患／胃腸障害	
	stomach and intestinal disorder
胃痛／腹痛	stomachache
一過性脳虚血発作	transient ischemic attack（TIA）
遺伝病	hereditary disease
胃の蠕動	stomach activity
いびき	snoring
異物感	foreign body sensation
胃壁	stomach wall
咽喉痛（喉の痛み）	sore throat
インフルエンザ	influenza／flu
う歯（虫歯）	cavity

エイズ	acquired immunodeficiency syndrome (AIDS)
炎症	inflammation
嘔気（吐き気）	nausea
黄疸	jaundice
嘔吐	vomiting
おたふくかぜ（流行性耳下腺炎）	
	mumps
おたふくかぜ・はしか・風疹	
	mumps／measles／rubella（MMR）
回復	recovery
かすみ目／霧視／視力低下	
	blurred vision
かぜ（普通感冒）	commom cold／cold
肩こり	stiff shoulders
合併症	complications
花粉症（枯草熱）	pollinosis／hay fever
がん	cancer
肝炎	hepatitis
癌腫	carcinoma
関節痛	arthralgia
感染症	infectious disease
肝臓病	liver disease
気管支炎	bronchitis
気胸	pneumothorax
急性腹症	acute abdomen／acute abdominal pain
狂犬病	rabies
狭窄	stenosis
狭心症	angina／angina pectoris

胸部痛	chest pain
虚血	ischemia
空気感染	airborne infection
くしゃみ	sneeze／sneezing
くも膜下出血	subarachnoid hemorrhage（SAH）
形成異常（奇形）	malformation
痙攣	spasm
けが／傷害	injury
血圧	blood pressure
結核	tuberculosis
月経異常／生理不順	
	irregular period
結石	calculus／stone
血栓	thrombus
血栓症	thrombosis
げっぷ	burp／belch
血餅／血栓	blood clot
血便	bloody stool
血流／血液循環	blood flow／blood circulation
下痢	diarrhea
眩暈（めまい）	vertigo／dizziness
元気がない／非活性	
	inactive
口渇／過度の喉の渇き	
	excessive thirst
高血圧	high blood pressure／hypertension
高血糖症	hyperglycemia
甲状腺疾患	thyroid disease
梗塞	infarction

紅斑	erythema
呼吸／呼息	breath
呼吸困難	dyspnea
骨折	fracture
COVID-19	COVID-19（coronavirus disease 2019）
コレラ	cholera
嗄声（声がれ）	hoarseness
痔／痔核	hemorrhoids
ジアルジア症	giardiasis
子宮筋腫／子宮平滑筋腫	
	uterine leiomyoma
歯茎出血	gums bleed
歯茎痛	gums pain
しこり	lump
歯痛	toothache
耳痛	earache
疾患	disease
湿疹	eczema
しびれ	numbness
ジフテリア	diphtheria
ジフテリア・百日咳・破傷風	
	diphtheria／pertussis／tetanus（DPT）
耳鳴	tinnitus
粥状硬化／アテローム性動脈硬化症	
	atherosclerosis
出血	hemorrhage／bleeding
術後合併症	postoperative complications
腫瘍	tumor
症状	symptom

用語集

食中毒	food poisoning
食欲不振	anorexia／loss of appetite
心雑音	heart murmur
滲出	oozing
心臓病	heart disease
腎臓病	kidney disease／nephropathy
心肺停止	cardiopulmonary arrest（CPA）
心不全	heart failure
蕁麻疹 じんましん	hives
水痘（みずぼうそう）	
	varicella／chicken pox
頭痛	headache
性感染症	venereal disease
咳／咳嗽	cough
赤痢	dysentery
石灰化	calcification
接触感染	contact infection
舌痛	sore tongue／tongue pain
喘息	asthma
蠕動／蠕動運動	peristalsis／peristaltic motion
前立腺肥大	prostatic hypertrophy
瘙痒（かゆみ）	itch（ing）
塞栓	embolism
体温	temperature
体重減少	weight loss
体重増加	weight gain
大動脈瘤	aortic aneurysm
唾液	saliva
だるい	feel heavy

痰／喀痰	phlegm／sputum
虫垂炎	appendicitis
腸チフス	typhoid fever
疲れやすい	tire easily
低血圧	hypotension
デング熱	dengue fever
動悸	palpitation
動静脈奇形	arteriovenous malformation（AVM）
疼痛	pain／ache
糖尿病	diabetes／diabetes mellitus
動脈硬化症	arteriosclerosis
突発性発疹	exanthema subitum
肉腫	sarcoma
日本脳炎	Japanese encephalitis
乳癌	breast cancer
妊娠	pregnancy
認知症	dementia
熱傷（やけど）	burns
熱性痙攣	febrile seizure
熱中症／熱射病	heat illness／heat stroke
捻挫	sprain
脳血管障害	cerebrovascular disorder（CVD）
脳梗塞	cerebral infarction
脳挫傷	cerebral contusion
脳腫瘍	brain tumor
脳卒中	(brain／cerebral) stroke／cerebral apoplexy
パーキンソン病	Parkinson's disease
肺炎	pneumonia

用語集

肺癌	lung cancer
梅毒	syphilis
排尿	urination／micturition
背部痛	back pain
白内障	cataract
破傷風	tetanus
発熱	fever
鼻水（が出る）	runny nose
パラチフス	paratyphoid fever
腫れ	swelling
皮膚炎	dermatitis
飛沫感染	droplet infection
肥満	obesity
百日咳	whooping cough／pertussis
貧血	anemia
風疹	rubella／German measles
不機嫌な（気分が変わりやすい）	
	moody
副作用	side effect
複視	double vision
腹痛	abdominal pain
腹部膨満感	abdomen feels swollen
不顕性感染／潜伏感染	
	latent infection
不正性器出血	irregular genital bleeding
不整脈	arrhythmia
普通感冒（かぜ）	common cold／cold
無菌性	sterility
不妊症	infertility

不眠症	insomnia
ふるえ	tremor
分泌	secretion
閉所恐怖症	claustrophobia
ペスト	plague
便	stools［大便］／urine［小便］
便秘	constipation
ほくろ	mole
発疹	rash
発疹チフス	epidemic typhus
ポリープ	polyp
ポリオ	polio
麻疹（はしか）	measles
マラリア	malaria
むくみ	swelling
胸の圧迫感	tightness in the chest
メジナ虫症	dracunculiasis
眼のかゆみ	itchy eyes
眼の病気	eye illness
卵巣嚢腫	ovarian cyst
流行性耳下腺炎（おたふくかぜ）	
	mumps
緑内障	glaucoma
淋病	gonorrhea

検査・処置・機器・医療用具など

RF 波（無線周波数）

radiofrequency

合図／指示	signal／instruction
核医学	nuclear medicine
ID カード	ID card
足跡	footprints
圧迫板	compressing plate
インターベンショナルラジオロジー	
	interventional radiology（IVR）
液体／水分	liquid／water
X 線	X-ray
X 線画像	X-ray image
X 線検査	X-ray test／X-ray examination
MRI（磁気共鳴映像法）	
	MRI（magnetic resonance imaging）
海草類	seaweed
貝類	shellfish
化学療法	chemotherapy
ガーゼ	gauze
画像	image／pictorial image
画像処理装置	（pictorial）image processing device
カテーテル	catheter
下部消化管 X 線撮影（注腸検査）	
	lower gastrointestinal tract radiography
	（lower GI）
カルテ	chart／clinical record／forms
鉗子	clamp
眼底検査	fundus examination／funduscopy／
	ophthalmoscopy
ガンマカメラ	gamma camera
機械／装置	machine／apparatus／equipment

ギプス	cast
胸部 X 線検査	chest X-ray examination
車椅子	wheelchair
下剤	laxative
血液検査	blood test
血管造影検査	angiography
検査	examination／test／exam
検査結果	result of the examination
検査台	examination table
高圧酸素療法	hyperbaric oxygen therapy（HBO）
抗原	antigen（Ag）
抗原抗体検査	antigen／antibody test
抗体	antibody（Ab）
氷枕	ice pillow
呼吸機能検査	lung function test／pulmonary function test
採血	blood collection／blood sampling
採尿	urine collection／urine sampling
座席／椅子	seat／chair
撮影伝票	medical form／voucher
殺菌	sterilization
三角巾	sling
シーツ	sheets
CT（コンピュータ断層撮影）	CT（computed tomography）
CT スキャン装置	CT scan device（apparatus）
シェル	shell
指示	instruction
磁石（磁気）	magnetic

手術用具	surgical instrument
紹介状	a letter of recommendation
消化器（X線）検査	
	digestive system examination／gastrointestinal（GI）tract X-ray（radiogram）
消毒薬	disinfectant
消毒用アルコール	rubbing alcohol
上部消化管X線撮影（胃透視）	
	upper gastrointestinal tract radiography（upper GI）
人工呼吸器	ventilator
診察券	hospital card
診察台	examination table
心電図	electrocardiogram（ECG）／［独］Elektrokardiogramm（EKG）
水薬／薬液	liquid medicine
ステント	stent
ストレッチャー（担架）	
	stretcher
SPECT（単一光子放射コンピュータ断層撮影）	
	SPECT（single photon emission computed tomography）
生理機能検査	physiological function test
造影剤	contrast medium／contrast agent
体温計	thermometer
注射	injection
注射器	syringe
昼食	lunch

超音波	ultrasound／sonogram
朝食	breakfast
聴診器	stethoscope
鎮痛剤／痛み止め	analgesic／painkiller
手すり	handrail
透視撮影台	fluoroscopy table
動注化学療法	arterial infusion chemotherapy／intra-arterial chemotherapy
動脈血酸素飽和度	arterial oxygen saturation （SaO_2）
トリアージ	triage
内視鏡	endoscope
内視鏡検査	endoscopy
軟膏	ointment
尿検査	urinalysis
脳波	electroencephalogram （EEG）
PACS（画像アーカイブおよび通信システム）	PACS （picture archiving and communication system）
発泡剤	effervescent granules
バリウム溶液	barium solution
バリウム嚥下造影検査	barium swallow test
バルーン	balloon
パルスオキシメータ	pulse oximeter
PCR 検査／ポリメラーゼ連鎖反応試験	PCR （polymerase chain reaction） test
HIS／病院情報システム	HIS （hospital information system）

病床	bed
氷嚢	ice pack
ピンセット／鑷子	forceps／tweezers
フィルムカセッテ	film cassette
フェイスガード	face guard
服薬指導	medication guidance
フラットパネル	flat panel
PET-CT（陽電子放射断層撮影・コンピュータ断層撮影）	
	PET-CT（positron emission tomography-computed tomography）
放射線	radiation
放射能	radioactivity
防腐剤	antiseptic
麻酔	anesthesia
松葉杖	crutch（es）
マンモグラフィ／乳房撮影	
	mammography／mammogram
綿棒	cotton swabs
モニタ	monitor
ヨウ素（沃素）	iodine
予防接種	vaccination
予約	appointment
予約票	reservation form
RIS／放射線科情報システム	
	radiology information system
レポート	report

所持品・衣服・装身具など

入れ歯	denture／artificial teeth／false teeth
クレジットカード	credit card
下着	underwear
ズボン	pants／slacks／trousers
スリッパ	slippers
装身具	ornament／accessories／jewelry
袖	sleeve
時計	watch
ネックレス	necklaces
ブラジャー	bra
ヘアピン	hair pin
補聴器	hearing aid
目隠し	blindfold
眼鏡	eyeglasses／spectacles

病院の部門・診療科・施設名など

~科／~部（病院部門名）
　　　　　　the Department of ~

アレルギー膠原病科
　　　　　　allergy and immunology

遺伝相談外来	genetic counseling clinic
医療相談室	medical care consultation room
受付	reception desk
栄養科	nutrition

栄養科・食事療法科
　　　　　　nutrition and dietetics

栄養指導	nutrition guidance
ATM	automatic teller machine
MRI 室	magnetic resonance imaging（MRI） room
エレベータ	elevator
会計／支払い	payments／accounting
回復室	recovery room（RR）
外来	outpatient department（OPD）
かかりつけ医	family doctor
核医学（RI）検査室	
	nuclear medicine room
眼科	ophthalmology
看護科	nursing department
看護相談室	nursing consultation room
冠疾患集中治療室	coronary care unit（CCU）
患者	patients
肝胆膵外科	hepatobiliary-pancreatic surgery
喫茶店	coffee shop
救急外来受付	reception desk of emergency room
救急室	emergency room（ER）
救急診療科／救急救命センター	
	emergency department／emergency center
胸部外科	general thoracic surgery
計算窓口	accounting desk
形成外科	plastic surgery／plastic and reconstructive surgery
外科	surgery
血液内科	hematology

健康診断	physical check-up
検査室	examination room／laboratory
更衣室	changing room
口腔外科	oral surgery
膠原病・リウマチ内科	
	rheumatology
公衆電話	public telephone
高度治療室	high care unit（HCU）
呼吸器内科	respiratory medicine／pulmonology
災害医療	disaster medicine
災害拠点病院	disaster base hospital
災害派遣医療チーム	
	disaster medicine assistance team
	（DMAT ディーマット）
産科	obstetrics（OB）
産婦人科	obstetrics and gynecology（OB／GYN）
CT室	computed tomography room
歯科	dentistry
歯科口腔外科	oral and maxillofacial surgery
自動販売機	vending machine
耳鼻咽喉科	otorhinolaryngology／ear, nose, and throat（ENT）
耳鼻咽喉科・頭頸部外科	
	otorhinolaryngology, head and neck surgery
集中治療室	intensive care unit（ICU）
主治医	attending physician
手術室	operating room（OR）
腫瘍科	oncology

用語集

腫瘍内科	medical oncology
循環器科	cardiology
消化器内科	gastroenterology
小児科	pediatrics（PED）
小児科・思春期科	pediatrics and adolescent medicine
小児外科	pediatric surgery
正面玄関	front entrance
食堂・カフェ	cafeteria
食道・胃腸外科	esophageal and gastroenterological surgery
腎・高血圧内科	nephrology and hypertension
神経内科	neurology（neuro）
診察	consultation／medical examination
診察室	consultation room／examination room
新生児室	neonatal room
新生児集中治療室	neonatal intensive care unit（NICU）
新生児治療回復治療室	
	growing care unit（GCU）
心臓血管外科	cardiovascular surgery
整形外科	orthopedics（ortho）
整形外科・スポーツ診療科	
	orthopedic surgery and sports medicine
精神科	psychiatry
総合診療科	general medicine／comprehensive diagnosis and treatment
大腸・肛門外科	colorectal and proctological surgery
タクシー乗り場	taxi stand／taxi stop
治験室	clinical trial room
低侵襲外科	minimally invasive surgery

トイレ	rest room／toilet room
糖尿病・内分泌代謝科	
	diabetes, endocrinology and metabolism
内科	internal medicine
内視鏡科	endoscopy
内分泌科	endocrinology
入院受付	inpatient reception desk
乳腺科	breast oncology
人間ドック	thorough medical exam／physical checkup
脳神経外科	neurosurgery
売店	stand／shop／booth
泌尿器科	urology
皮膚科	dermatology
病院	hospital
病棟	ward
病理科	pathology
病理診断科	diagnostic pathology
福祉相談室	welfare consultation room
婦人科	gynecology（gyn）
分娩室	delivery room（DR）
ペインクリニック	pain clinic
放射線科	radiology
放射線腫瘍科	radiation oncology
放射線治療室	radiotherapy room
麻酔科	anesthesiology
麻酔科・ペインクリニック科	
	anesthesiology and pain medicine
夜間受付	night-reception／night reception desk

用語集

薬剤部／薬局	pharmacology／pharmacy
薬局	pharmacy
輸血科	transfusion medicine
リハビリテーション科	
	rehabilitation medicine
臨床検査科	laboratory medicine

memo

memo

memo

memo

memo

謝　辞

Acknowledgments

Thank you for your great cooperation.

Mr. Kenneth Maynor，Mrs. Cheryl Maynor，中島美和 氏，倉持 徹 氏，木暮陽介 氏，Suero 尊子 氏，芳士戸治義 氏，その他多数の外国人患者様たち，編集に携わっていただいた小枝克寿 氏，高柳ユミ 氏をはじめとする方々の協力と示唆をいただき，本書の刊行に至ったことを感謝いたします．

Yasuaki Sakano

—— 著者略歴 ——

坂野康昌

順天堂大学 保健医療学部 診療放射線学科
副学科長・特任教授

1976 年 千葉大学医学部附属診療放射線技師学校卒業，同年診
療放射線技師免許取得，1985 年 明治大学法学部法律学科卒業，
2012 年 首都大学東京大学院博士前期課程修了，修士（放射線
学），2018 年 首都大学東京大学院博士後期課程修了，博士（放
射線学），東京都立荏原病院・広尾病院・駒込病院で放射線技
師長，都立病院放射線統括技師長を務め，首都大学東京客員
教授，つくば国際大学医療保健学部診療放射線学科教授・学
科長などを歴任，2019 年より現職．2013 年に叙勲，瑞宝双光
章を受章．

診療放射線技師のための医療英語

2021 年 4 月 15 日　1 版 1 刷　　　　　　　　　©2021

著　者
　さかの　やすあき
坂野康昌

発行者
株式会社 南山堂　代表者 鈴木幹太
〒 113-0034　東京都文京区湯島 4-1-11
TEL 代表 03-5689-7850　　www.nanzando.com

ISBN 978-4-525-02261-7

A0226110101-A

透視台（X線TV）などにおける指示

装置に上がって／装置の隣に立って背中をつけてください.

> Step your feet on the apparatus and lean your back on it.
>
> Stand right next to the apparatus and lean back.

台が水平まで動きます.

> This apparatus will begin to move down horizontally.

最初の位置は仰向けです.／仰向けに寝ていてください.

> First position is lying on your back.

次に，少し頭が下がりますので，横の棒を持ってください.

> Next, it will slightly move down, please hold on to the side handrails.

右体を左に約30度斜めに持ち上げます.

> Lift your right body to the left in a slanting position at about 30 degrees.

右に30度ほど斜めに向けてください.

> Try to turn to your right about 30 degrees in a diagonal position.

仰向けに寝てください.
(supine position – lie on your back)

> Please lie on your back.

右を下／左を下にして寝てください.
(lateral position – lie on your side)

> Please lie on your right / left side.